Planning for Library Services to People with Disabilities

ASCLA Changing Horizons Series , Number 5

Rhea Joyce Rubin

Association of Specialized and Cooperative Library Agencies

American Library Association

Chicago 2001

Published by the Association of Specialized and Cooperative Library Agencies
American Library Association
50 East Huron Street
Chicago, IL 60611

ISBN 0-8389-8168-2

The paper used in this publication meets the minimum requirements of American National Standard for Information Sciences—Permanence of Paper for Printed Library Materials. ANSI 239-48—1992.

Printed in the United States of America.

05   04   03   02   01   5   4   3   2   1

CONTENTS

Appendices

For Photocopying
  (No page numbers appear on these pages)
    Library Scan: Planning for Library Services for People with Disabilities
    Additional Questions for Academic, School, and Special Libraries
    User and Non-User Survey: Planning for Library Services for People
       with Disabilities
    Planning Process Budget Worksheets

ACKNOWLEDGMENTS

Massachusetts Advisory Committee Members

Filippa Marullo Anzalone, School of Law Library, Northeastern University
Kim L. Charlson, Braille and Talking Book Library, Perkins School for the Blind
Marylyn Howe, Massachusetts Assistive Technology Partnership
James Izatt, Talking Book Library, Worcester Public Library
Sandra Lindheimer, Middlesex Law Library, Trial Court of Massachusetts
Mary Rose Quinn, Saugus Public Library

Massachusetts Scan and Survey Instrument Pretest Sites

Porter Memorial Library, Blanford, MA
Springfield Technical Community College
Berkshire Law Library, Pittsfield, MA
New Bedford Free Library
Morse Institute Library, Natick, MA
Maxwell Library/ Bridgewater State College

Massachusetts Board of Library Commissioners Staff

Shelley Quezada, Consultant

California Readers

Alan Bern, Berkeley Public Library
Marti Goddard, San Francisco Public Library

The development of this process was supported in whole or in part by the Institute of Museum and Library Services. However, the opinions expressed herein do not necessarily reflect the position or policy of that agency, and no official endorsement should be inferred.

Funding for the original project was from the Massachusetts Board of Library Commissioners with grant monies from the federal Library Services and Technology Act (LSTA).

FOREWORD

By Shelley Quezada, Consultant,
Library Services to the Unserved,
Massachusetts Board of Library Commissioners

Under the requirements of the Library Services and Technology Act, the *Massachusetts Long-Range Plan (1998-2002)* identified the need for libraries to be more responsive to people with disabilities. Although the Americans with Disabilities Act (ADA) has been law for more than ten years, the state library agency (the Massachusetts Board of Library Commissioners or MBLC) was concerned that many residents with visual, hearing and mobility impairments were unable to fully utilize libraries. Based on surveys and focus groups, it was determined most libraries in the state had not addressed the issue. They neither had adaptive equipment for a range of disabling conditions nor were their staffs trained to meet the needs of these consumers.

In April 1999, the Board engaged the services of Rhea Joyce Rubin to develop a streamlined planning process based on her work as one of the principal trainers of *Planning for Results,* a 1998 Public Library Association training. Given her extensive experience in helping libraries serve the disability community, she was asked to design a planning process specific to issues of serving people with disabilities and to provide training in its use. Over the course of several months Rubin met with an advisory group representing different types of libraries as well as members of the disability community to discuss drafts of three surveys that libraries would administer as part of their pre-planning efforts. Public, academic and special libraries field-tested a variety of community/library/user scan instruments. It was concluded that, given the challenges of serving people with disabilities, only libraries which had already completed a long-range plan would be encouraged by MBLC to take on the specialized requirements of this new planning process. The final document was written so that all types of libraries – public, school, academic, and special – would find it relevant and useful.

In November 1999, the MBLC offered a series of three-day workshops by Rubin to introduce staffs to the completed document, *Planning for Library Services for People with Disabilities: A Process for Libraries in Massachusetts.* Workshop attendees participated in immersion exercises and listened to a panel of disabled consumers who communicated their frustration in using libraries before being introduced to the mechanics of the planning process per se. This training helped prepare library staffs to begin planning efforts in their own communities and alerted them to a special MBLC Mini-Grant round for projects up to $20,000 for those who successfully completed a draft planning document. The mini- grant served as an incentive for libraries by providing an opportunity to purchase adaptive workstations, provide special signage, outfit a meeting room with a sound system, purchase specialized materials, or respond to specific needs identified in their draft plan of service.

In July 2000, 12 libraries – including a hospital and prison library – received approval for special project funding based on objectives outlined in their plan. Later that year another group – including two university libraries – participated in training and made a commitment to apply for grant funds. Undoubtedly this planning document has made a critical difference for libraries seeking to offer better services and programs but unsure of the steps that they needed to take. *Planning for Library Services for People with Disabilities* has provided a process that enables library staffs to negotiate the complex but necessary task of expanding library services to all members of their community.

INTRODUCTION

Another Planning Process?

This ten-point process has been designed to work in conjunction with an already existing library plan. Because of the currency and popularity of *Planning for Results* (Public Library Association, 1998), many libraries have recently written long range plans. Others used the previous PLA model, *Planning and Role Setting for Public Libraries* (1987).

Both of these models highlight the selection of priority clusters of services – these were called *roles* in the earlier process and *service responses* in the new version. Although the roles or service responses could be tailored for a specific target group, few libraries have adapted them to services for people with disabilities.

Some libraries have used generic long-range planning processes or amalgams of these approaches to develop plans that resulted in general goals and objectives often broken down by age group. Rarely have libraries concentrated on meeting the needs of people with disabilities in their plans of service. This process allows a library to design a plan with the needs of people with disabilities in mind. The new plan will fit within its existing larger long-range plan.

The library is asked first to assess its own collections, services, policies, and facilities and then to survey its community of people with disabilities. A planning committee is convened to identify issues facing the population of people with disabilities. Next the library examines its current plan of service to see how it can be rewritten or augmented to ensure that is addresses those issues. After looking at available resources and prioritizing possible services, the plan is written.

The order of the process – steps one through ten – is not sacrosanct. A library that has already done some planning regarding people with disabilities can start at the appropriate part of this process to complete its plan. For example, a library with a good ADA advisory committee can ask that group to serve as the planning committee. Or a library that has done an ADA self-assessment survey as part of a building renovation plan can skip some or all of the library scan.

The new plan will:

- ensure that all parts of the larger plan are inclusive
- add objectives and activities of special interest to people with disabilities based on identified issues

- guarantee that library services are available on an equal basis to all members of the community
- attract people with disabilities to use the library
- position the library as an information access point for people with disabilities, their relatives, and their service providers

Why A Special Plan for People with Disabilities?

21% of the US population – more than one in every five people – has a disability as defined by the Americans With Disabilities Act. A disability is a condition or disease that limits a person's ability to perform one or more major life activities such as communicating, hearing, eating, walking, or working. In the United States, an estimated .6% of the population are blind, 3% are visually impaired, 5% have speech or language impairments, 2.9% have mobility impairments which require them to use wheelchairs or other devices, .6% are deaf, 8% are hearing impaired, 15% have learning disabilities, 5% have developmental disabilities, 2% have mental retardation, and 5.5% have severe mental illness. (Please see the glossary for definitions of these terms.) Note that these numbers add up to more than 21 because many people with disabilities have more than one limitation.

It is important to note that disability rates vary greatly by ethnicity. Native Americans have the highest rate of disability for any racial or ethnic group, 23.9%. When examining the rate of disability of adolescents and working age adults, the difference is even greater; the overall rate of disability for Americans aged 15 to 64 is 18.7% while the Native American rate for that age group is 27.1% African-Americans have the second highest rate of disability, 21.6%. The difference is starker when rates of severe disability are used. Blacks have the highest rate of severe disability at 12.7%; 9.9% of all Americans have severe disabilities. People of Hispanic origin have a disability rate significantly lower than the national average: 16% as compared to 21%. And the disability rate for Asian and Pacific Islanders is even lower: 12% as compared to the national 21%. The reasons for the differences in disability rate include genetics and social factors such as comparative income levels, availability of health insurance, and educational levels.

The proportion of the US population with disabilities has risen markedly during the past twenty-five years, according to the National Institute on Disability Research and Rehabilitation. There are three primary reasons for this. The first is our aging population. The likelihood of having a physical or sensory disability increases with an individual's age. According to the census information, older adults experience disability at twice the rate of those in older working ages (45-64) and four times the rate of younger working ages (18-44). Since the average age in our country is rising, the number of people with one or more disabilities will continue to grow. A side result of the growing proportion of our population who are older than 65 is that the overall population with disabilities is increasingly influenced by the disability rate among older adults.

The second reason for the increase in people with disabilities is an increased proportion of youth with disabilities (since so many more at-risk babies are saved) and better diagnosis and reporting of their disabilities. Among children, there have been increases in the prevalence of asthma, mental disorders such as attention deficit disorder, mental retardation, and learning disabilities. Among young adults, rates of orthopedic impairments, nervous and mental disorders are on the increase.

The third reason for the growing disability rate is the rapid increase of population among minority groups. As discussed above, some ethnic minority groups which have grown considerably in the past decade also have especially high rates of disability.

When projecting rates of disability for the future, all of these trends need to be considered. Two other factors affecting the prevalence of disability are social and economic conditions and immigration. There is a higher rate of disabilities among people in areas that are less affluent and where educational attainment levels are low, and among new immigrants from countries with poor health care.

By definition, all of these people with disabilities need one or more accommodations to ensure their ability to use the library building and/or library resources. Libraries need to plan to provide both physical (or architectural) and intellectual or (programmatic) access.

But the issue of library service to people with disabilities is more complex than just ensuring that current services are accessible; often people with disabilities have additional or different information needs based on their disability or on their economic and educational profile. People with disabilities are, on average, less educated, less employed, and poorer than other Americans. For example, the poverty rate of working age people with disabilities is 40%. Another factor is that people with disabilities are less likely to have a computer and/or use the Internet than others. A 1999 National Telecommunications and Information Administration survey found that only 25% of Americans with disabilities aged 15 or older own computers and that only 10% ever access the Internet. All of these facts point to special information needs and library assistance.

The Americans with Disabilities Act (1990) is a broad civil rights act which guarantees that all people, regardless of disability, have full access and participation in society. Two of the ADA's mandates are especially significant for libraries. First, *any* public library must provide equal services to *any* person requesting them, regardless of disability. The ADA states that "*No* qualified individual with a disability shall, by reason of such a disability, be excluded from participation in or be denied the benefits of the services, programs, or activities of a public entity, or be subject to discrimination by any such entity." (ADA, Section 202, italics added.) Second, programs and services for people with disabilities must not be segregated. Every public entity must "administer services, programs, and activities in the *most integrated setting* appropriate to the needs of qualified people with disabilities." (56 Federal Register 35719, italics added.)

On July 26, 1999, the ninth anniversary of the ADA, President Clinton stated that the three core principles of the government's disability policy are inclusion, independence, and empowerment. "We must infuse the values of the ADA – equality of opportunity, full participation, independent living, and economic self-sufficiency – into all aspects of government and social policy…Now we endeavor to empower individuals with disabilities with the tools they need to achieve their dreams." In many cases the library, the keeper of information and knowledge, has those tools and must make them available to all.

What Are We Undertaking?

Before beginning this planning process, your library administration needs to consider a number of questions:

- Who will be responsible for the planning process? Although as many staff as possible should be involved in some aspect of the planning, one or two people should be appointed to manage the process from beginning to end. The library's ADA Coordinator is an appropriate person for this assignment. If the library has a planning officer or similar position, that person and the ADA Coordinator might collaborate. In some libraries, a public service librarian with a special interest in disability or a Board member with a concern about inclusiveness might be asked to be responsible.

  - How long will the process take? Depending on the library's internal schedules and staffing patterns and the availability of the person assigned the responsibility, the process will take from three to six months.

  - What are we promising? By surveying the community and then convening an advisory committee, the library is committing itself to providing some new services or programs for people with disabilities. These may be minor revisions to current procedures and policies or brand new offerings. If the library administration is not willing to make some changes in the status quo and to insist that staff will endorse and implement those changes, the planning process should not be undertaken.

1. GATHER INFORMATION

The first step in any planning process is to gather information that will serve as a baseline for discussion about the library's possible futures. In planning for services to people with disabilities this means assessing the library's current resources, finding out about the population of people with disabilities in the library's community, and surveying library users and non-users with disabilities.

In the following pages you will find three pre-tested survey instruments for you to use in gathering relevant information. (At the end of the manual are clean masters of the instruments for you to duplicate.) The first is the library scan which asks about your library's current compliance with the ADA and its staff training, collection, services, and assistive technology. The library scan is the easiest to do because all of the information requested should be kept in some fashion by the library already. If your planning is for a multi-type system or region, each member library should complete the form.

The second instrument is the community scan which asks for current information and projections on the local population of people with disabilities. The library researches how many people with each of seven specific disabilities live in the service area, their ages, and their employment or education. This information is extremely important because disability is not a monolithic condition; in order to plan for services the library must know exactly which disabilities are most prevalent. If your community has a predominance of people who are deaf you may wish to begin with or concentrate on services to them; such services are completely different than services to people who are blind or have mental illness. In addition to data on the population, the community scan requires information on other agencies, organizations, and libraries that serve people with disabilities in your community.

The community scan is time consuming and may be frustrating for a number of reasons. First, most libraries do not have this information at hand and do not collaborate with agencies and organizations which do. Second, each agency (e.g. school district, department of vocational rehabilitation) collects and keeps its data its own way, using its own terminology and age categories, so that often the numbers are not comparable. (See the appendix on *Disability Statistics and Terminology* for more on this.) Some of the alternative terms and categories are mentioned on the scan instrument; more are included in the glossary. Use whatever terms and categories make sense in your situation.

Keep in mind that the purpose of the community scan is to develop a picture of your community in terms of disabilities, not to create an elegant and perfect statistical record or to gather data comparable to other communities. The information you gather is for your own planning purposes only. The best advice on this is: persevere! The knowledge you gain will be invaluable. To assist you in this, the appendix has lists of resources you can consult. If it is impossible to find local statistics, you can extrapolate from the national numbers provided.

The third information-collecting instrument is a survey of library users and non-users. Using the contacts you've made completing the community scan, identify the types of people you want to survey. Rather than trying to survey people with all seven types of disabilities right now, you may choose to survey two in this planning cycle and the others in the next. For example, if your area has more people with learning disabilities and with mental retardation – and fewer resources for them – than you had realized, you might target the survey to those two populations. Then, with the help of local agencies and organizations, distribute the survey to as many individuals as possible to determine their experiences using libraries in the past, any barriers to using your library services, and their other information access points. Note that this is not a user satisfaction survey but a data-gathering instrument.

SCANNING THE LIBRARY

HOW TO DO THE SCAN

The designated ADA Coordinator for your library should already have the information requested in the library scan. If not, answering the questions on the attached form will assist him/her in fulfilling the ADA Coordinator role.

Here are some tips for completing the scan:

- Complete the library scan first, then do the community scan before doing the user survey.

- If you are planning for people with disabilities as a multitype library system, consortium, network, or region, consider having each member library complete the form. All the scans can then be collated to give an overall picture of the library resources of the system or region.

- See the glossary for an explanation of the terms used in the scan.

- See additional questions for school, academic, and special libraries on page 19.

- Use additional pages as necessary to complete the library scan.

- If you need information on physical accessibility (questions #1 and #2), see the *ADA Accessibility Guidelines* available in print from the US Department of Justice or online at http://www.access-board.gov/adaag/html/adaag.htm Library Buildings, Equipment and the ADA (ALA 1996) may also be helpful. Note that the *ADA Accessibility Guidelines* are being revised; a new edition will be available in 2000.

- If you need information on making your website accessible (question #14), see any of these for advice. Accessibility Guidelines Page Authority http://www.w3.org/TR/WAI-WEBCONTENT or Adaptive Technology Resource Center http://www.utoronto.ca/atrc/ or Designing a More Useable World http://www.trace.wisc.edu/world/ or Bobby http://www.cast.org/bobby/.

Library Scan: Planning for Library Services for People with Disabilities

1. Does your library comply with the ADA regarding physical accessibility to and within the library facility? Mark Y for yes and N for no.

    ____ Parking spaces
    ____ Ramps and curb cuts
    ____ Building and interior entrances (doors)
    ____ Stairs, floors, and elevators
    ____ Stack aisles
    ____ Reading/study area aisles and seating areas
    ____ Service counters
    ____ Desks and other furniture
    ____ Telephones
    ____ Drinking fountains
    ____ Alarm systems
    ____ Signage
    ____ Bathrooms

2. Does your library have a plan to come into compliance with the ADA by fixing those items marked N?

3. Who is your library's ADA Coordinator?

4. Does your library have an advisory group of people with disabilities?

5. Does your library have any staff members with disabilities? If so, what disabilities?

Please continue on next page

     Rubin

6. *Does your library offer staff ongoing training in the following areas? Mark* Y *for yes and* N *for no.*

    _____ Sensitivity training on disabilities
    _____ Customer service for people with disabilities
    _____ How to be a sighted guide for blind patrons
    _____ Sign language basics
    _____ Local agencies and organizations to whom you can refer people with disabilities
    _____ Awareness of special equipment and its availability? (assistive technologies)
    _____ How to use the equipment and to assist others in using it
    _____ Federal and state laws concerning services to people with disabilities

7. *What alternative format materials does your library own? Check all that the library has.*

    _____ Large print books
    _____ Audio books/books on tape (commercial)
    _____ Talking books (NLS)
    _____ Braille books
    _____ Print/Braille books
    _____ Closed caption videos
    _____ Described videos
    _____ Instructional videos on sign language
    _____ Toys and other tangibles
    _____ Adaptive technology for loan
    _____ Other (please specify)

8. *What special services are offered to patrons with disabilities? Check all that are offered.*

    _____ Extended loan periods
    _____ Extended reserve periods
    _____ Library cards for caregivers/proxies
    _____ Ability to check out more than the usual number of materials
    _____ Dial-in access to the OPAC
    _____ Electronic access to library resources from home (or dorm)
    _____ Home delivery service
    _____ Books-by-mail
    _____ Brochures and library maps in alternative formats
    _____ TTY reference service

Please continue on next page

_____ Fax access to reference and/or circulation desk
_____ E-mail access to reference and/or circulation desk
_____ ASL or realtime captioning offered at public programs
_____ Volunteer reader in library
_____ Volunteer technology assistant in library
_____ Radio reading service or Newsline for the Blind
_____ Other (please specify)

9. What assistive technology (non-computer) does the library offer? Check all the library has.

_____ Public use TTY/TTY payphone
_____ Assistive listening devices for use in the library
_____ Assistive listening system in meeting rooms/auditoriums
_____ Hand-held magnifiers for in-library use
_____ Electronic magnifiers (CCTV)
_____ Reacher/grabbers
_____ Wheelchairs/scooters for in-house use
_____ Talking signage
_____ Photocopy machine with large print capability
_____ Adjustable lighting with magnification
_____ Other (please specify)

10. Does staff know how to use all the items checked above?

11. Does the library have adapted computer workstations?

12. If so, what adaptations do the workstations have? Please check all that you have:

_____ Wheelchair height table/carrel
_____ Adjustable height table/carrel
_____ Screen enlarger device (magnifier)
_____ Text magnification software
_____ Screen reader (voice output software)
_____ Text to speech software (reading software)
_____ Voice recognition system (voice input software)
_____ Thought organization software

Please continue on next page

_____ Braille printer
_____ Large print printer
_____ Alternate keyboards
_____ Mouse alternatives
_____ Touch screens or overlays
_____ Scanners (OCR)
_____ Switches and switch software
_____ Pointing and typing aids
_____ Other (please specify)

13. *Does staff know how to work all of the checked features?*

14. *Does your library have a Web page? If so, is it accessible? If you are not sure, take the Bobby test at* http://www.cast.org/bobby/

Additional Questions for Academic, School, and Special Libraries

1. Do you have reserve collections in alternative formats? Check all that are available.

_____ Audio tape
_____ Computer disk
_____ Large print
_____ Braille
_____ Access to the Perkins School Service
_____ Other (please specify)

2. Do you have recommended/required reading collections in alternative formats? Check all that are available.

_____ Audio tape
_____ Computer disk
_____ Large print
_____ Braille
_____ Access to the Perkins School Service
_____ Other (please specify)

3. Is the campus/school district testing center in your facility? If so, what accommodations are offered for people with disabilities?

4. Is there an on campus office that provides services for people with disabilities? If yes, what are the hours of operation?

5. Does the campus office for disability services provide any services within the library to library users? If yes, what?

Please continue on next page

6. Who provides direct assistance to people with disabilities using the library?
Check all that apply.

       ____ Patron's personal assistant
       ____ Staff from another agency/department
       ____ Trained volunteers from another agency/department
       ____ Library staff
       ____ Trained library volunteers

7. What are the hours these assistants are available?

SCANNING THE COMMUNITY

HOW TO DO THE SCAN

Completing the community scan will take some staff time and effort but will bring many rewards. The results will be informative and provide you with much new information that you can use in everyday tasks as well as in long range planning.

Here are some tips for completing the scan:

- Do the community scan second; begin with the library scan and end with the user survey.

- Consider doing the community scan as a collaborative staff effort. For example, seven staff members may research the community, each looking at one specific disability group. One person (perhaps the ADA Coordinator) should be designated as the coordinator of all the information gathered; this person is responsible for completing the scan forms.

- See the glossary for terms used in the scan.

- Note that each data-collecting agency uses its own terminology and age categories. This makes it extremely difficult to compile information from different agencies. (See the appendix *Disability Statistics and Terminology* for more on this.) Some of the alternative terms and categories are mentioned on the scan instrument; more are included in the glossary. Remember that the purpose of the community scan is to develop a picture of your community in terms of disabilities, not to create an elegant and perfect statistical record or to gather data comparable to other communities. Use whatever terms and categories make sense in your situation.

- All questions apply to non-institutionalized civilian individuals. If you have a residential facility for people with disabilities in your area, note those statistics also.

- Whenever possible, use local statistics. (See appendices for resources). If you cannot find local statistics, use the national formula given to determine an estimated number for your area. Sources of formulas appear in the glossary.

- Note that if you add all the statistics together you will have far more than 21% of your population with disabilities. This is because many people with disabilities have more than one impairment.

- If you cannot find the age-breakdown statistics requested in question 2, simply skip over that question to the next. The local school district is a good source for numbers regarding school-age children as they are required by law to maintain statistics. The local area agency on aging may keep statistics on the over 65 age segment.

- Answer the scan questions based on the primary community of users for your library. The first step is to define your primary community of users. For example, a public library has its local citizens as its primary users; non-residents may be the library's secondary users, and the users of other libraries in your region or network may be your tertiary users. In a law school library, the law school students and faculty are the primary users; students and faculty of other colleges within the university are secondary, and the general public and consortium members are tertiary.

- If you are using the community scan for a multitype library system, consortium, network, or region, consider having each member library complete the form for its primary community of users. All the scans can then be collated to give an overall picture for the system or region.

- Use additional pages as necessary to complete the community scan.

Community Scan: People with Disabilities

1. How many people with disabilities live in your service area? (Use relevant, current local statistics if possible; if these are not available use the nationally based formula given to determine an estimated number for your area.)

A. People who are blind or are severely visually impaired?
    Source Used:
    (US formula is 3% of population)

B. People with speech or language impairments?
    Source Used:
    (US formula is 5% of population)

C. People with mobility or orthopedic impairments, including wheelchair users?
    Source Used:
    (US formula for mobility impairments is 2.9% and for wheelchair users it is .4%.)

D. People who are deaf or hard of hearing?
    Source Used:
    (US formula is 4.4% of population)

E. People with learning disabilities?
    Source Used:
    (US formula is 15% of population)

F. People with developmental disabilities or mental retardation?
    Source Used:
    (US formula is 1.8% of population)

G. People with severe mental illness or serious emotional disturbances?
    Source Used:
    (US formula is 5.5% of population)

Please continue on next page

2. What are the ages in this population?

A. People who are blind or are visually impaired?
  School age (6 to 16, 18, or 22 years)
  Adult (16 or 18 to 64 years)
  Older Adult (65 years and older)
  Source:

B. People with speech or language impairments?
  School age (6 to 16, 18, or 22 years)
  Adult (16 or 18 to 64 years)
  Older Adult (65 years and older)
  Source:

C. People with mobility or orthopedic impairments, including wheelchair users?
  School age (6 to 16, 18, or 22 years)
  Adult (16 or 18 to 64 years)
  Older Adult (65 years and older)
  Source:

D. People who are deaf or hard of hearing?
  School age (6 to 16, 18, or 22 years)
  Adult (16 or 18 to 64 years)
  Older Adult (65 years and older)
  Source:

E. People with learning disabilities?
  School age (6 to 16, 18, or 22 years)
  Adult (16 or 18 to 64 years)
  Older Adult (65 years and older)
  Source:

F. People with developmental disabilities or mental retardation?
  School age (6 to 16, 18, or 22 years)
  Adult (16 or 18 to 64 years)
  Older Adult (65 years and older)
  Source:

Please continue on next page

G. People with severe mental illness or serious emotional disturbances?
    School age (6 to 16, 18, or 22 years)
    Adult (16 or 18 to 64 years)
    Older Adult (65 years and older)
    Source:

3. What percentage of students enrolled in the local school district have disabilities? In the local community college? Other colleges and universities?

    Sources:

4. What percentage of people in the total community of people with disabilities is employed? (Use relevant, current local statistics if possible; if these are not available use the National Organization on Disability's 1998 figure of 29% to determine an estimated number for your area.)

    Source:

5. What local agencies and organizations provide services to this population?

A. People who are blind or are visually impaired?

B. People with speech or language impairments?

C. People with mobility or orthopedic impairments including wheelchair users?

D. People who are deaf or hard of hearing?

E. People with learning disabilities?

F. People with developmental disabilities or mental retardation?

G. People with severe mental illness or serious emotional disturbances?

6. What other libraries are there in your geographic area which serve people with disabilities?

SURVEYING USERS AND NON-USERS

HOW TO DO THE SURVEY

Using the contacts you've made completing the community scan, identify library users and non-users to survey. Most agencies and groups will not give out the names of their clients or members, but may be willing to distribute the survey on your behalf.

Here are some tips for implementing the survey:

- Your goal is to get as many responses as possible. Advertise the survey by placing signs near the reference and circulation desk and by sending notices to local newspapers and to other agencies and organizations' newsletter. To further publicize the survey, you may want to insert a large print bookmark about it into every book checked out.

- Consider having service desk staff distribute the survey to any library user with an obvious disability or whom you know has a disability because of special services you already provide. But do not ask patrons "Do you have a disability?" to avoid causing embarrassment.

- If your library has a website, add the survey – or an announcement of its availability.

- You may need to translate the survey and have it available in other languages.

- Don't forget to survey kids. You can reach children and youth through schools as well as community agencies. In the case of young children, ask for a parent to complete the survey.

- If you are doing this as a mail survey, be sure to include a cover memo specifying a date (one to two weeks later) by which it should be returned and thanking the recipient for participating. (A sample cover memo follows). Enclose either a self-addressed envelope marked "Free Matter for the Blind" for blind recipients or a stamped self-addressed envelope.

- The survey itself is in large type. Be prepared to create the user survey in braille, audio, and electronic formats if requested. This is essential so that it can be used by a broad array of people with disabilities.

- If you need assistance preparing the alternative formats or in implementing the survey, call your local State Library or Talking Book Library.

- If your library is considering the purchase of adaptive equipment, you may want to add a list of possible purchases and ask "Please check off which of the following you would like to have at the library." This instrument does not include a generic list of possibilities so as not to raise unreasonable expectations.

Sample Cover Letter for Survey

Thank you for sharing your experiences using our public library. This survey is also available in braille, audiotape, and electronic computer disk. Please call [name] at [(xxx) xxx-xxxx] to request a copy of they survey in an alternative format.

Please return the survey by [date] in the enclosed pre-addressed stamped *(or "free matter for the blind")* envelope.

Thank you again for completing the survey so that we can improve our services to people with disabilities.

User and Non-User Survey: Planning for Library Services for People with Disabilities

Note: This survey is available in alternative formats (braille, audio, and electronic). Please request the version you would like.

1. If you use the library, when did you use it last?

2. In what way(s) does your disability make it difficult to use the library? Check all that apply.

      ___ transportation to library
      ___ parking at library
      ___ physical access to and within building
      ___ hours open
      ___ communication with staff
      ___ attitudes of staff or public
      ___ inability to find or reach library materials
      ___ inability to use library materials
      ___ difficulty using the computers
      ___ other (please specify)

3. Which library services do you use or would you like to use? Check all that apply.

      ___ information and referral
      ___ check out materials
      ___ read newspapers and magazines
      ___ children's services
      ___ Internet and database searching
      ___ programs and events
      ___ other (please specify)

Please continue on the next page.

4. What could the library provide to assist you in using the library's materials and services?

    ___ books by mail
    ___ extended loan periods
    ___ reference services by fax or TTY
    ___ alternative formats of materials (specify)
    ___ different technology (specify)
    ___ help finding books
    ___ other assistance from staff
    ___ other (please specify)

5. Have you requested these materials/services in the past? If so, were they provided to you? If not, what reason was given?

    ___ Yes   ___ No

    Reason:

6. Have you ever used a computer or other equipment at the library?

    ___ Yes   ___ No

7. Did you already know how to use it?

    ___ Yes   ___ No

8. Were you given instructions or help?

    ___ Yes   ___ No

9. What could we do to make the computer workstations easier for you to use?

10. Do you have access to a computer at home or at work?

    ___ Yes   ___ No

    If so, is it

    ___ Macintosh   ___ IBM compatible

Please continue on the next page.

11. If you have a computer at home or at work, what adaptive equipment or software do you use?

12. What service agencies besides the library do you use for information and referral?

13. How do you find out about programs and services at the library?

14. How can the library best communicate with you in the future?

15. What is your disability? (optional)

16. Please mark your age range:

    ____ 6-12 years old
    ____ 13-22
    ____ 23-65
    ____ 66 and older

17. Are you currently in school? If so, at what level?

    ____ Elementary school
    ____ High school
    ____ Community college
    ____ University
    ____ Post graduate

Please continue on the next page.

17. If you have completed your education, please specify the extent of your schooling.

       ___ Elementary school
       ___ High School
       ___ GED
       ___ Community college
       ___ University
       ___ Post graduate degree

18. Are you currently employed?

       ___ Yes   ___ No

       If yes, ___ Part time   ___ Full time

19. Other comments (please use back of sheet):

Thank you for completing our survey!

2. CONVENE A PLANNING COMMITTEE

An advisory committee is essential for any planning process which purports to be responsive to the community. By convening – and listening to – a group of concerned community members the library ensures that its plan is in tune with real needs and concerns. That, in turn, guarantees more use of any new services and programs and more support for the plan and for the library.

Besides being politically astute, building your plan on the community's stated needs means that budget requests are grounded in something larger than internal projections. For example, instead of requesting funds for "100 more picture books because of estimated losses from the collection" a library might request funds "to develop a collection of materials for caregivers of children with multiple disorders."

An ideal advisory committee is large enough to represent the community yet small enough to work together. A group of 12 to 18 is probably best. But there is no magic number; since representation of the community is most important, let that determine the committee's size. Good committee work can be done with as many as 30 people using the procedures described in the next chapter.

Of course, the *composition* of the advisory committee is key. You want to invite

- people with each kind of disability found in your community
- caregivers (family or paid) of people with disabilities
- members of organizations of people with disabilities
- staff of other agencies which serve people with disabilities
- special education directors
- representative(s) of other libraries in the area doing more or different programs and services for people with disabilities
- library staff representatives

Don't forget to involve youth (or their advocates), adults, and older adults as you select individuals from each of the six categories listed above.

Be sure the individuals you select are stakeholders and true representatives; that is, they are knowledgeable, connected and vocal people who have a reason to be concerned with the outcome of your work, who will make real contributions to the planning process, and will advocate for the resulting plan. In addition, committee members should be able and willing to devote their time and expertise to the library.

When you invite a person to participate on the advisory committee, send a letter in the appropriate format (i.e. large type, audio recording, braille, or electronic) which explains why you selected him or her, the purpose of the committee, how long the planning process will last, how many meetings are anticipated, and your expectations for their involvement. Then follow up with a telephone call.

Typically you are asking a committee member to attend one all day meeting (approximately six hours including lunch) and one three hour meeting as well as to read and comment on drafts. You may want to have a third meeting at the end of the process also. The time span will be anywhere from one to six months depending on the library's staffing and internal scheduling.

Once a person has agreed to be on the advisory committee, send her/him the findings of the community and library scan in preparation for the retreat. Ask for feedback on the community scan, especially if you have had to rely on statewide or national demographics. Even within a state, areas vary greatly in the number of people with disabilities and the types of disabilities represented. Also ask for projections; for example, are there any reasons to think that the number of people with disabilities will increase or decrease significantly during the next five years?

If you have never worked with people with disabilities, try to educate yourself before you convene the committee. (See tips sheets in the appendix for introductory information.) Be aware that meeting planning may be more complex than usual in that you will probably need to provide anything in writing in multiple formats, depending on the individuals' needs. You may also have to have interpreters or captioning at the meetings and, of course, all meetings will have to be held in fully accessible locations.

After the plan is complete and formalized, be sure to send copies of the plan to the committee members, asking them to distribute them to everyone they know. Then send a personalized thank you to each member and his or her employer if that is relevant.

PLANNING PROCESS BUDGET WORKSHEET

Category	Number	Unit Cost	Cost
Committee Support			
Photocopies	_____	_____	_____
Braille transcription	_____	_____	_____
Audiorecording	_____	_____	_____
Postage	_____	_____	_____
Other	_____	_____	_____
Meeting Costs			
Room rental	_____	_____	_____
Refreshments	_____	_____	_____
Technology	_____	_____	_____
Interpreter fees	_____	_____	_____
Facilitator fees	_____	_____	_____
Facilitator travel	_____	_____	_____
Other	_____	_____	_____
Staff Costs			
Overtime	_____	_____	_____
Substitutes	_____	_____	_____
Temporaries	_____	_____	_____
Other	_____	_____	_____
Publishing Plan			
Desktop publishing	_____	_____	_____
Graphic artist	_____	_____	_____
Braille transcription	_____	_____	_____
Audio recording	_____	_____	_____
Other	_____	_____	_____
Other	_____	_____	_____
	_____	_____	_____
	_____	_____	_____
	_____	_____	_____
Total		$_____	

3. IDENTIFY ISSUES

The first meeting of the advisory committee is an exciting and significant event which sets the course for the plan. The daylong meeting is devoted to identifying issues of importance to the population of people with disabilities and deciding which issues the library should address. As in *Planning for Results*, the library's possible goals and activities are not discussed until after this first meeting.

Recognizing key issues is not as simple as it sounds. Often you will not get thoughtful responses if you ask a person "what issues do you face?" You can better shed light on significant issues by encouraging a discussion on the positives and negatives of the current situation as well as the opportunities and threats to the community. This is called a SWOT exercise; details on how to have such a discussion follow below.

Tips for Planning the Issues Meeting

1) Libraries which have the resources to do so are encouraged to hold the meeting as a "retreat" away from the library's basement meeting room and in a nicer setting. Sometimes a local country club or membership organization will loan a facility for the day. By meeting off-site, library staff can avoid inevitable work distractions. Also, a retreat setting usually makes the meeting special so that advisory committee members realize that their participation is valued.

2) Have a designated facilitator. If you can hire a professional, fine; if not, you may find a community volunteer with facilitation skills. Or ask a library staff member who is especially adept at running meetings. Whoever the facilitator is, that person's job all day should be process only and not content.

3) Food is an excellent motivator and also serves as a thank you to your committee members who have agreed to spend a day sharing their expertise and opinions.

4) Prepare the meeting room so that each committee members' special needs are addressed. For example, you may need an amplification system, a projection system for real time captioning, and/or a sign language or oral interpreter.

5) Arrange the room with separate tables (round are best) for every 5 to 6 people. Have a flipchart easel and pad by each table. For each table provide a recorder (either a staff person, a member of the Friends of the Library, or a volunteer). Seat each group of 5 or 6 members so that the type of participants at each table are mixed. (For example, a youth with a physical disability, an older

adult with hearing loss, a mobility instructor for newly blinded people, an outreach librarian, and a deaf adult may share one table).

6) Note that anything written on flipcharts during the day must also be read aloud so that blind, visually impaired, and learning disabled people can participate fully.

7) Even if the agenda is progressing more slowly than expected, do not skimp on breaks. Instead lunch can be shortened to one-half hour or discussion can continue as people eat unless you are using interpreters and/or realtime captioners who also need a break.

Sample Agenda for 6 Hour Advisory Committee Meeting of 12-30 People

9:00 All participants are welcomed. Library director (or staff person responsible for planning process) explains the library's current planning status (i.e. this is to be an add-in to an existing plan that was written in 1998). "Housekeeping" information is shared (i.e. location of bathrooms, availability of coffee and snacks). Introduction of facilitator who describes the day's agenda and sets ground rules for communication (e.g. one person speaks at a time).

9:15   Self-introductions at each table

9:30   Report on community scan findings (by person responsible)

9:40   SWOT Exercise

11:00 Coffee Break

11:15 Identify Issues

12:30 Lunch Break

1:30   Prioritize Issues

1:45   Select Issues the Library Might Address

3:00   Adjourn

Procedure for SWOT Exercise (Strengths, Weaknesses, Opportunities, and Threats)

- Ask each group to concentrate first on the present situation in your town, college, or area by discussing the following question. "As a person with disabilities or a person who works with people with disabilities, what are the main *strengths* of this town (or attending this school or college)?" Allow 15 -

20 minutes for discussion with the recorder making notes on flipchart paper. Examples of strengths may be the proximity to an Assistive Technology Center or an excellent special education department in the public schools.

- Now ask each group to continue discussing the present with the question "As a person with disabilities or a person who works with people with disabilities, what are the area's *weaknesses*? That is, what are the main disadvantages of living in this town (or attending this school or college)?" Allow 15 - 20 minutes for discussion with the recorder making notes on flipchart paper. Examples of weaknesses may be the distance from a large city or lack of good paratransit.

- Next ask: "What *opportunities* exist in our town (school or college) for improving life for people with disabilities? " Again allow 15 - 20 minutes for discussion with the recorder making notes on flipchart paper. Examples may be a new industry opening offering job opportunities or a new elected official with a concern for people with disabilities.

- Continue with the question "What *threats* are there to people with disabilities in our town (school or college)?" Once again allow 15 - 20 minutes for discussion with the recorder making notes on flipchart paper. Examples may be growing reliance on expensive electronic communications or destruction of inexpensive housing.

- During the coffee break, post every chart with all answers to a question grouped together. With the assistance of the recorders, combine any identical or overlapping responses, noting the number of duplicates.

- After the break reconvene as one large group. Ask the recorders to read aloud the answers to each question, reporting the number of duplicates.

- Check to be sure that everyone (including you!) understand all the posted answers.

- Explain to the group that similar answers that appear in two or more areas usually point to significant issues. Based on this, note the issues which have surfaced. For example, technology may appear as both an opportunity and a threat. Or, moving the state school for the deaf out of the area may be listed under both opportunity and threat.

- List the identified issues on a new flipchart. Read the list aloud.

- Check with the participants that the list is realistic and fairly comprehensive. If necessary, add issues.

Procedure for Prioritizing Issues

- Probably there are more than six issues listed, so it is necessary to prioritize down to a workable list of six or fewer. Ask the group to vote for the most *important* issues. Spend a few minutes defining "important" as having the most impact, consequence, and immediacy. *Impact* means "How basic is this issue? How many other things depend on this?" *Consequence* mean "How good or bad will it be if we don't address this issue?" *Immediacy* means "How urgent is this? Can dealing with it be postponed?"

- Have the participants vote either by raising hands or by placing sticky colored dots on the flipcharts next to the six they consider most important. (Note that if you use sticky dots some participants may need assistance; the recorders can be asked to help as needed.)

- Read aloud the issues that have the most votes (or stickers). If there are fewer than six which got a preponderance of votes, fine. Otherwise, take the top six. These are now the issues to consider for library response.

Procedure for Selecting Issues For the Library to Address

- Explain to the participants that the last task of the day is to consider which issues the library might best respond to. Library administration and staff will decide *how* to respond later as they are the experts on library collections and services and know the library's resources and capabilities. But since the committee is most familiar with other programs for people with disabilities, the library wants their opinions on which issues are most suitable for the library to address. The library might be a key player, a partner agency, or a supporter of the efforts of other effective groups.

- Taking each issue one at a time, ask the group as a whole to discuss the following questions:

    - Are other agencies or organizations working on this issue?
    - If yes, might they be interested in collaborating?
    - If no one is working on it, why not? Who should be working on it?
    - Is there a part of the issue that the library seems particularly well suited to address?
    - Does the library have resources that are critical to dealing with this issue?

- Now you have a list of one to six critical issues which the library seems suitable to address. Quite an accomplishment for one long day's work!

4. ANALYZE THE LIBRARY'S CURRENT PLAN

The second meeting of the planning committee should be held as soon as possible after the retreat to keep up the momentum. This meeting will focus on the fourth part of the planning process.

It has two steps. First you will check that your current plan of service is inclusive of people with disabilities. Second you will see if the issues selected by the advisory committee are already addressed in the library plan; if not, additional goals and objectives will be added to the existing plan.

1. Examine your library's current long-range plan. Turn to the mission statement or list of priorities or directions and implementation plan to assess them from the point of view of patrons with disabilities. For example, here's the Anytown Public Library's mission statement: "The Anytown Public Library provides information about popular cultural and social trends; general information and answers to questions; curriculum support for students in K-12 schools; support for personal growth and development; and information services for the business community."

According to that mission statement, the first two priorities in the Anytown Public Library's plan are information services. In planning for serving people with disabilities, Anytown Library must check that its implementation plan to provide information services addresses such issues as:

- Providing answers in non-print formats
- Allowing for questions from people who cannot get to the library and/or cannot use a telephone
- Providing longer loan periods for people who cannot get to the library
- Capable staff trained on disability issues

For each part of your library's mission statement or plan for service, ask the following questions:

- Are our facilities *architecturally accessible*?
- Do we have the appropriate alternative *formats* of materials for people with disabilities?
- Does our *collection* address the information needs of people with disabilities?
- Do we have alternative *modes of access* to this program or service?
- Do we need an enhanced or extended *service* or a special *program* to ensure that people with disabilities are included?

- Do the library *policies* related to this goal provide for special needs?
- Is *staff* trained in providing this service or program for people with disabilities?
- If *technology* is involved, do we have accessible equipment and adaptations needed for people with disabilities?

If the answer to any question is "no," an additional objective or activity should be written for that goal in the plan. To continue with the Anytown example, the information services goals may need the addition of "provide fax reference services (incoming questions and outgoing answers) upon request."

It may not be clear to the library staff what objectives or activities will meet the needs inherent in your negative answer to one of the above questions; this is one place where the expertise of advisory committees is invaluable. For instance, ask "How could we best provide people with disabilities with answers to questions they might ask the library? What formats are easiest to use?" The committee will have suggestions to make the library more inclusive.

2. The second step in this part of the planning process is to compare the issues identified at the retreat with your current plan. For instance, you may decide that the second priority in Anytown Library's plan addresses the identified issue of "Need for better information services for families of children who have learning disabilities." In that case, use the eight questions above to ensure that the general information goal of the library will really cover the information services specified in the committee's issue.

If one of the identified issues from the advisory committee's retreat is "Lack of city agency staff able to assist people with disabilities," nothing in Anytown Library's plan fits. In this case, an additional goal or an objective to the information services goal must be added to the library plan specifically on this issue. Again, the committee has the expertise to advise you on the contents of the goal. (Note that the actual writing of the goals will be covered in the next chapter and will be done by library staff).

At this point you also need to return to the results of the community scan and the user/non-user surveys. Your new goals and objectives should relate to those findings as well. If they do not, you need to consider writing yet another new goal or objective.

5. DRAFT GOALS AND OBJECTIVES

Goals are statements of where you want to be. Objectives are ways of getting there. A personal goal might be to buy a new car; one objective is to "find" the money to buy it. (Note that the "how" of finding the money – perhaps save for it, perhaps earn extra money – is not the objective but an activity.) A library's goal might be to provide all citizens (students) with an excellent print and non-print collection, the latest information technology, and a well-trained and welcoming staff. Objectives for this goal include selecting the materials and technology and training the staff.

This sounds simple, but each planning process presents its own method of constructing goals and objectives. If your library has used *Planning for Results* (*PFR*), you have written goals which do not mention the library. Instead the emphasis is on the library user. For example "Small business owners in Anytown will have the information they need to succeed." The formula for writing such a goal is "who benefits + the benefit + the result." In the Anytown example, who benefits are the small business owners; the benefit is having information; and the result is successful business.

In *PFR*, objectives are how the library will measure its progress toward reaching a goal. The formula for writing such an objective is "what + desired change + time frame." For the Anytown goal above, an objective might be "During FY 2000, the use of the library's small business information Web page will increase by 15%." Another objective might be "At least 75% of businesspeople using the Anytown Library's business collection during FY 2000 will indicate that they found the information they needed to make informed decisions."

If your library has used *Planning and Role Setting for Public Libraries* (*PRSPL*), you have written two types of goals: service goals and management goals. Service goals are written from the point of the view of the user. An example is "Members of the community are able to obtain materials and services to pursue their own learning and meet their individual information needs." A *PRSPL* objective for this example might be "To increase adult attendance per capita for programs related to self improvement by 25% during FY 2000. *PRSPL* management goals are written from the point of view of the library. For example, "The library recruits, trains, and retains the most competent personnel available." An objective might be "To increase the number of full-time professional staff to eight by the end of FY 2000."

Other planning processes suggest still other ways of writing goals and objectives. The main difference is that in some approaches the objectives include the "how." In the Anytown example, an objective might be "During FY 2000, the library will install two CD-ROM business databases." But in both *PFR* and *PRSPL*, the "hows" are included in the activities or actions rather than the objective.

No matter which planning process your library has used, it is essential that the goals identify priority areas for the library and the community and provide the foundation for objectives which are measurable and allow you to measure progress toward the goal. Write your goals and objectives for service for people with disabilities in the same style your current plan is done.

As you write, keep in mind that there are three types of measures to consider:

- *Number of people served.* You can count the total number of users who use a service each time they use it (counting total users) or you can count the person only once regardless of how many times he or she uses it (counting unique individuals served.)
- *How well the service meets the needs of the people served.* You ascertain the users' opinions about how well the library met their needs. These opinions could be about the quality, value, satisfaction, or even the impact of the service.
- *Total units of service provided by the library.* You count the number of actual library service transactions that were done to make progress toward a specific goal. These include the standard library output measures such as circulation, reference interactions, and programs offered.

6. DETERMINE AVAILABLE RESOURCES

Before goals and objectives can be finalized, and an implementation plan designed, your library's resources need to be considered. Does the library have sufficient resources to cover any revisions or new goals and objectives created in the previous parts of this process?

First you must estimate what resources will be needed to accomplish the new or revised goals and objectives. For each objective, calculate the necessary:

- staff time
- specialized skills or expertise
- books and other materials
- technology or equipment
- facilities or space
- supplies and materials

Next, the library administration needs to consider the requirements you have listed for the new or revised goals in light of current resources. Usually at least some of the resources are available but others are not. Questions include:

- Does the library have enough *staff* to do this?
- Does the library staff possess the *skills* needed to do this?
- Does the library own the *collections* or have access to the materials needed to do this?
- Does the library have the *technology* or equipment needed to do this?
- Does the library have the *facilities* or space needed to do this?
- Does the library have the supplies and *materials* needed to do this?

Once you have determined the gaps between what is available and what is needed, the administration must consider methods of finding resources. Reallocation of current resources is an obvious consideration. For example, if space is the issue, changing the layout of the building might help or rescheduling other activities might work. If reallocation will not cover the needs, other possible solutions can be discussed. Is there another way to get what is needed? In the space example, alternatives include finding free program space elsewhere in the community or renting a space. To take another example, if staff expertise is an issue, partnering with another agency or organization with that knowledge and experience might work. Or inviting an expert agency to train current library staff. Of course, finding additional funding to purchase resources is always a possibility, too. Perhaps grant money or local business support is available.

The convener of *Planning for Library Service for People with Disabilities* should be included in resource allocation discussions to help balance the library's current situation with the needs identified by the advisory committee. For example, if resources are scarce it may be necessary to narrow the focus of an objective (e.g. tailoring the objective to children only or to one disability group only). Perhaps the most difficult phase of any planning is deciding what is equitable for the community as well as reasonable for library staff and resources.

7. FINALIZE GOALS AND OBJECTIVES

Now that resource decisions have been made, it is time to revisit the goals and objectives and refine them as necessary. You may even have to eliminate one or more, though ingenuity usually allows for retaining the goal in a smaller scale or narrower focus.

As you are revisiting the goals and objectives, pull out the original community scan and the issues identified by the advisory committee and consider these questions:

- Can the library address this issue more efficiently by partnering with another agency or organization?
- Can the library simply assist another agency or organization which has a similar goal?
- Can the library postpone implementing this goal until the next budget or planning cycle?
- Can the goal be retained if the objectives are rewritten on a smaller scale?

And while you're rethinking the goals, ask two basic questions:

- Is this goal achievable and measurable?
- Does this goal truly address the issue raised by the community scan or the committee?

8. DRAFT PLAN

Finally it is time to draft the plan! It should include the following pieces:

- An introduction explaining the purpose of the plan and the process used
- Acknowledgements of the advisory committee members and all staff who contributed
- Goals and objectives
- Activities
- Implementation (or action) plan

The introduction and acknowledgments are best written by one person, probably the person designated as the coordinator for the planning process. But the activities should be written by a group of library staff who may be involved in implementing them and who have knowledge of the library's internal strengths and weaknesses.

Activities are things the library will do to satisfy the objectives. Depending on how the goals and objectives are written, activities may be developing actual products (e.g. offering programs, installing an assistive listening system) or they may be more specific tasks necessary to create products (e.g. finding speakers for programs or researching assistive listening systems). If your activities are the broader type, you will also want to list the tasks in the implementation plan.

Assuming that you are poised to write broad activities, the easiest way to start is for the staff group to brainstorm alternatives to fulfill your objectives. Start by reminding everyone of the goal and then, taking one objective at a time, ask "How can we do this?" Some possibilities include providing information resources, producing programs, training staff, collaborating with other groups. Be as creative as possible and leave the practicalities aside for the moment.

Once you have a long list of potential activities, select the ones that will have the most impact on the goal. Do this by asking the group these questions:

- Which activities will be most effective in helping the library meet the goal?
- Which are most likely to excite current and potential users?
- Which build on staff competencies and interests?
- Which have the best chance of successful completion?
- Are adequate resources available?

Narrow your list to approximately four activities per objective. Don't lose any of the group's good ideas though; some of the activities might work for another objective or might be deferred to the next planning cycle.

At this point, distribute the draft goals, objectives, and activities to the advisory committee for feedback. A meeting of the committee at this point is optional.

While waiting for the committee members' responses, staff can begin on the last section, the *implementation plan*. This is sometimes called an action plan. Usually produced as a chart, the action plan lists each objective (broken down by activity and specific tasks) with the person responsible for its implementation, a date for completion, and the measures of success. Note that checking each measure (e.g. number of people using new adaptive technology) is an activity with its own tasks.

9. FINALIZE THE PLAN

Finalizing the plan includes getting any necessary approval(s), publishing, and distributing the plan. Often the activities and the implementation plan are not included in the final plan but are considered internal documents. This gives the library flexibility in revising assignments and timetables as necessary.

From whom do you need to *obtain approval*? Of course, the library administration must agree to the plan. In most libraries, the Board of Commissioners or another official body must approve any plans with financial implications. The library administrator should determine who needs to authorize it

Publishing the plan means producing it in one or more editions for the library board, other city agencies, and the public. For example, you may print the entire plan – with graphics and an attractive cover – as well as an abbreviated version on a bookmark . Don't forget to have the plan available in accessible formats also.

Ask your advisory committee to help *distribute* the plan so that it gets to as many people in your target populations as possible. Have the key points printed in the local newspaper as well as in newsletters for people with disabilities, for relevant agencies and organizations, and for caregivers.

10. EVALUATE

No discussion of planning can ignore evaluation. The two are like sides of a coin, inseparable.

Before you begin implementing your new plan, consider evaluation. If your objectives are well-written they include the measures you will use to evaluate them. Each measure should be noted on the implementation plan so that checking on the objective's status is easy to do throughout the cycle.

Whoever is responsible for the overall coordination of a specific goal should do a monthly assessment. The following questions should be asked for each activity:

- Is it on schedule?
- Have there been any problems with completing this activity?

If all is well, congratulate the person responsible for the activity and move on. If the activity is behind schedule, ask:

- Why is it off track?
- What can be done to bring it up to speed?
- What resources are lacking?
- Does the implementation plan need revisions because of this delay?
- What impact does this delay have on other activities?
- On achieving the objective?
- On achieving the goal?

There should be no surprises at the end of the planning cycle. "Oops! We never did that!" indicates poor planning and poorer assessment. To assist in future planning, a final evaluation of the planning itself should be done at the end of the cycle. You may want to involve the planning committee in your evaluation of the process. For each goal, answer the following questions:

- How did this goal assist in fulfilling the library's mission?
- To what extent did this goal provide a basis from which staff could write clear and measurable objectives?
- Should this goal be maintained as written, revised, or dropped?

For each objective answer the following questions:

- Did this objective help fulfill the goal?
- Was this objective successfully met?

- If not, why not?
- Were the activities successful?
- Were the allotted resources (staff, collections, technology, facilities, materials) sufficient?
- What lessons were learned during implementation of this objective which could inform future planning?

Of course, the ultimate evaluation is from the users' point of view. If possible, survey users (and their caregivers, parents, teachers, etc.) as to their satisfaction with the library's innovations and their suggestions for future changes.

GLOSSARY OF TERMS

Note: Please see the appendix on disability statistics and terminology for a discussion of the conflicting definitions and complex data gathering in the field of disability.

ADA   Americans with Disabilities Act. Public Law 101-336. A civil rights law passed in 1990 to ensure equal opportunities for people with disabilities. The law covers employment, public services and accommodations (including libraries), transportation, and telecommunications relay.

ALD   Assistive listening device. Usually refers to an aid for one-to-one communication. Hearing aids and cochlear implants are personally-owned ALDs. Other devices are owned by agencies – such as libraries – for use on-site. These usually have a microphone worn or held by a speaker which transmits sound directly to a receiver being held or worn by a person with hearing loss.

ALS   Assistive listening system. Usually refers to aids for group communication, for example in meeting rooms or auditoriums. They may be permanently installed or portable. The two major types, both of which can work in conjunction with existing public address systems, are infrared systems and FM systems. Also known as "Wide Area Assistive Listening Systems."

ASL   American Sign Language. A manual communication system using gestures and hand symbols. Based on concepts, rather than words, ASL is recognized as its own language, not a translation of spoken English. ASL is the fourth most common language used in the US because it is considered the native language of people who are born deaf, grow up with deaf parents, and/or are educated at schools for the deaf.

Adaptive technology   Technology which allows a person with a disability to be self-sufficient. Most often used in reference to personal computers which have been modified to accommodate a specific disability. For the purpose of libraries, it covers any device or equipment which allows an individual to work or gain access to information independently.

Assistive technology   Standard term used by federal programs for adaptive technology. (See above). Assistive technology is any product or piece of equipment which makes life easier for a person who has a disability or chronic illness. These devices may range from a simple gripper for a person with arthritis to a custom voice-activated computer for a person without use of his/her arms.

Blind A person who, after correction by glasses or surgery, has visual acuity of 20/100 or less in her/his better eye; or (if visual acuity is greater than 20/200), a peripheral field of vision of 20 degrees or less. According to the US Census, .6% of residents are blind and another 3% are severely visually impaired.

Books on Tape Current terminology for cassette recordings of books, previously called audio books or audio cassettes. Refers to commercially produced spoken word recordings rather than talking books from the Library of Congress network of libraries.

Braille A tactile reading and writing system, invented in 1829, consisting of raised dots produced in a six-dot configuration which represents the alphabet and certain letter combinations and word contractions. Used by approximately 85,000 people (a small proportion of blind people), particularly those who are born blind and/or are educated at schools for the blind. For these people, Braille is often the format of choice for reading because of its portability, its ability to allow the reader to review, and its non-reliance on electronics.

CCTV Closed circuit television print enlargement device. Also called electronic magnifiers or video print magnifiers. Telesensory's *Aladdin* magnifiers and Optelec's *Clearview* magnifiers are popular examples.

Closed caption videos Videos which include a hidden print subtitle of the spoken script. Designed for deaf people and people who are heard of hearing, these videos are also often helpful for people learning English. In order to see the captions, a closed caption decoder must be used. Libraries often label these videos with a "CC" symbol.

Closed caption decoder Device which reveals the captions on closed caption videos. Most televisions and VCRs now have these devices built in due to a 1990 law requiring them in TV sets (with screens larger than 13") by 1993.

Communication disorders People with communication disorders include individuals who are deaf or hard of hearing, or who have speech, voice or language disorders.

Deaf A person who is deaf is unable to rely on audition alone to understand speech; s/he must also rely on visual and other cues. Deafness can be caused by accidents, medication, illness, or hereditary conditions. As used in this process, the deaf population includes two major groups: people who consider themselves part of a cultural group with ASL as their distinct first language and people referred to as "late-deafened" who lose their hearing after having acquired language fluency. "Hard of hearing" refers to people who may be born with residual hearing or who experience a hearing loss later in life. According to the U.S. Census, .6% of the country's population is deaf and another 8% is severely hearing impaired.

Described videos Videos which incorporate narration, describing the key visual elements such as setting and action for viewers with visual impairments. The narrator's voice is heard during pauses in the video's regular dialogue.

Developmental disabilities A severe, chronic disability attributed to a mental and/or physical impairment that is manifested before the individual is eighteen years old and is likely to continue indefinitely. Such disabilities substantially limit at least three major life activities such as self-care, receptive and expressive language, learning, mobility, self-direction, and/or independent living. Included are mental retardation, autism, spina bifida, cerebral palsy, cystic fibrosis, epilepsy, muscular dystrophy, fetal alcohol syndrome and other neurological conditions acquired in childhood. Because early federal definitions equated developmental disability and mental retardation, the two terms are still often used synonymously – and incorrectly – by the public. In fact people with developmental disabilities can have exceptionally high IQs; an example is Stephen Hawkings, a physicist and author who has ALS ("Lou Gehrig's Disease"). According to the Association of Retarded Citizens, 5% of Americans have developmental disabilities, and only 58% of those individuals have mental retardation.

Disability A disability is a condition or disease that substantially limits a person's ability to perform one or more major life activities such as communicating, hearing, eating, walking, or working. According to the ADA, the term "disability" includes orthopedic disorders, mental retardation, mental illness, speech and hearing disorders, perceptual dysfunction, visual impairment, specific learning disabilities, HIV, and other diseases and conditions. According to the latest census information, approximately 21% of Americans have disabilities. Note that "disability" and "impairment" are not identical as impairments do not necessarily require significant limitations in human activities. See more on this in the appendix "Disability Statistics and Terminology."

Emotional disorders *see Mental Illness*

Handicap The World Health Organization defines a handicap as "the loss or limitation of opportunities to take part in the life of the community on an equal level with others" resulting from "cultural, physical or social barriers which prevent their access..." So the handicap is not the disability but a result of the greater community's barriers to people with disabilities. Note that most disability organizations do not use the word "handicap" or "handicapped" at all, considering it a derogatory description of a person's limitations which has been replaced with the term "disabled."

Hard of hearing or hearing impaired People who may be able to hear and understand some speech but have difficulty decoding the spoken word without assistance and cannot use hearing as a major means of receiving information.

According to the US Census Bureau, 8.6% of the country's population is deaf and severely hearing impaired. The Center for Disease Control estimates that another 10% of adults – primarily older adults – have some hearing loss (are hard of hearing).

Individuals with Disabilities Education Act (IDEA) Federal legislation passed in 1994 requiring students with special needs to be integrated as fully as possible into regular classrooms and to be assisted according to their individual needs. One result of the IDEA is that school districts keep detailed statistics on disability.

Large print Text printed in fourteen point or higher as compared to nine point which is the standard size for book publishing. Most commercially produced large print books are printed in sixteen point which is approximately one-sixteenth of an inch high; twenty-four point is approximately one-eighth of an inch high. Also referred to as large type.

Late deafened *see* Deaf

Learning disabilities Disabilities which make it difficult for individuals to process and/or interpret sensory information. The area of difficulty is typically very specific; an individual usually has little trouble learning in areas other than the one affected. Over 100 different specific learning disabilities have been identified; the most commonly known is dyslexia, which affects a person's ability to read. According to the National Institutes of Health, 15% of Americans have learning disabilities. Note that Attention Deficit Disorder (ADD) and Attention Deficit Hyperactivity Disorder (ADHD) are not considered learning disabilities although an estimated one-third of children with learning disabilities also have ADD or ADHD.

LSTA Library Services and Technology Act. Federal aid to public libraries distributed as a grant program through the state libraries.

Mental disability Classification used by the US Census Bureau for people who report "the existence of mental retardation, Alzheimer's disease, senility, dementia, learning disabilities, or any other mental or emotional condition."

Mental disorder Preferred by the American Psychiatric Association, this term is synonymous with the more commonly used term "mental illness." It does not assume a disease with treatable symptoms as does the word "illness" and includes both organic and functional disorders.

Mental Illness or Emotional Disorders Mental and emotional illnesses are disturbances of thought, feeling, or action leading to illogical thinking, irrational thoughts, and/or delusions. The most prevalent disorders are depression, manic-depressive illness, schizophrenia, and anxiety disorders (such as panic disorder, obsessive-compulsive disorder, post-traumatic stress disorder). "Serious" mental illness (SMI) refers to chronic mental illness which is disabling. According to the National Institute of Mental Health, 15% of the country's population has some degree of mental illness and 5.5% have serious mental illness or emotional disturbances that cause dysfunction.

Mental Retardation The most common form of developmental disability, mental retardation refers to significantly subaverage intellectual functioning resulting in or associated with impairments in adaptive behavior. An IQ of under 70 usually delineates mental retardation. According to the Association of Mental Retarded Citizens, 1 to 3% of the US population has mental retardation in one of the four major classifications: mild, moderate, severe, or profound. 87% of people with mental retardation have mild or moderate retardation; only 13% have severe or profound retardation, defined as an IQ under 55.

Mobility impairments Disorders that affect an individual's ability to move. Also referred to as orthopedic disorders. Included are spinal cord injuries and musculoskeletal disorders (MSD). Spinal cord injuries are catastrophic and usually permanent injuries leading to severe disabilities. MSD is a broad category of conditions which affect soft tissue and/or bone, causing alterations in structural integrity and resulting in pain, altered function and/or disability. The most common MSD are osteoarthritis, rheumatoid arthritis, tendonitis, and lower back injury. According to the National Center for Health Statistics, 2.9% of people in the U.S. have serious mobility impairments and .4% of Americans use wheelchairs.

Motor impairments People with motor impairments are also called "physically disabled" and may have impaired mobility or reduced use of other muscle groups. For example, some people with motor impairments may use wheelchairs while others may not be able to speak and or to use their hands.

NLS National Library Service for the Blind and Physically Handicapped. A service of the Library of Congress, providing books on record and tape and in braille directly to print handicapped individuals via the mail through a network of state and local talking book libraries.

OPAC Online Public Access Catalog. The automated version of a card catalog. May also be known as a PAC, public access catalog.

Orthopedic disorders *see* Mobility Impairments.

People with Disabilities Term which replaces "handicapped people;" note the "people first" language. According to the ADA, a person with a disability is anyone who has a physical or mental impairment that substantially limits one or more of the person's major life activities; has a record of such impairment; or is regarded as having such an impairment. According to the 1990 census information, approximately 21% of Americans have disabilities.

Print disabled A term used in the library profession for people who cannot use standard print text no matter the cause. May include people with temporary limitations as well as permanent ones.

Psychiatric disorders Synonym for mental illness, this term includes schizophrenia, affective disorders, and anxiety disorders. Not all people with psychiatric disorders are considered disabled because the disorders may not interfere with daily life activities.

Reading machine A stand-alone machine which includes a scanner, word recognition software, and a speech synthesizer so that printed materials can be "read aloud." May include a computer that can then store, manipulate, and print the materials which are read aloud. The Kurzweil Reading Machine was the original, followed by the *Kurzweil Personal Reader* (KPR). Telesensory's *Reading Edge*, the *Kurzweil 1000*, and Arkenstone's *VERA* are other popular examples.

Realtime captioning A method which displays the spoken word as it is spoken. It allows a person who is deaf or hard of hearing to read printed text as it is spoken aloud by another. The speech is input into a court reporting stenography machine or into a regular computer and text is immediately displayed on a computer monitor (for private viewing) or projected onto a larger screen (for public viewing). This method is especially valuable for people with difficulty hearing who do not know ASL. Sometime referred to as CART for Communication Access Realtime Translation or Computer Aided Realtime Translation.

Refreshable braille A braille display of computer data which allows the data on the computer screen to be read by a blind person. A device with a row of electronic simulated braille cells, each of which is represented by six or eight pins. These pins are raised or lowered by the computer which translates the keyed-in letters into braille. As the braille is read, it is continually changed (or refreshed) to the next letter or word.

Screen reader *see* Talking Computer

Sensory disorders A category of disorders which describes impairments in receiving or transmitting of the senses: sight, hearing, taste, smell, and touch.

Specific Learning Disabilities *see* Learning Disabilities

Speech disorders Correctly known as speech, voice, and language disorders, these affect a person's ability to speak in an understandable fashion without assistance. Such disorders affect approximately 5% of the US population according to the American Speech-Language-Hearing Association. Speech disorders include motor or neurogenic disorders caused by diseases of the central nervous system such as Parkinson's disease; articulation or phonological disorders such as lisping, usually of unknown cause; and fluency difficulties such as stuttering. Voice disorders may affect pitch and can be caused by overuse, misuse or abuse of the voice and by diseases such as cancer. Language impairments, including aphasia or loss of speech, may be caused by developmental disabilities, hearing impairments, traumatic brain injury, or stroke.

State Library A state agency, established to provide research services for the Governor, officers, and legislators; to provide library services to state government, and to provide consultation and/or services to libraries and systems.

Talking computer A personal computer equipped with both the hardware (a speech synthesizer) and software (a screen reading program) so that the words on the computer monitor – for example the library's catalog – are "read aloud" by the computer.

TDD Telephone device for the deaf. Also known as a text telephone or TTY. (See below).

TTY Teletype device for the deaf. Also known as a TDD or text telephone. Provides a print display of the telephone conversation, allowing direct telephone communication by deaf people. "TTY" is the term of choice in the deaf community; "TDD" is seen as a term developed and used by hearing people.

Visually impaired People who, though not legally blind, cannot use conventional print media. Can be caused by the process of aging itself. In libraries, visually impaired people and blind people are sometimes jointly referred to as "print disabled." According to the U.S. Census Bureau, 3.2% of Americans are visually impaired (but not blind) despite prescription eyeglasses.

Wheelchair users People who use wheelchairs have limited mobility due to the absence, paralysis, or other impairment of the limbs, or to chronic disease. According to the National Center for Health Statistics (from the National Health Interview Survey) .4% of the American population use wheelchairs.

APPENDICES

Bibliography on Planning

Bolt, Nancy and Sandy Stephan. *Strategic Planning for Multitype Library Cooperatives: A Planning Process*. Chicago: American Library Association, 1998.

Himmel, Ethel and William James Wilson. *Planning for Results: A Public Library Transformation Process*. Chicago: American Library Association, 1998.

Jacobs, M.E.L. *Strategic Planning: A How-to-Do-It Manual for Librarians*. NY: Neal-Schuman Publishers, Inc., 1990.

Markuson, Carolyn and others. *School Library Media Center Long-Range Planning Guide: A Workbook for Massachusetts School Library Media Centers*. Boston: BiblioTech Corporation for the Massachusetts Board of Library Commissioners, 1999.

McClure, Charles R. and others. *Planning and Role Setting for Public Libraries*. Chicago: American Library Association, 1987.

Nelson, Sandra. *The Concise Planning for Results*. Chicago: American Library Association, 2001.

Van House, Nancy A. and others. *Output Measures for Public Libraries*. 2d ed. Chicago: American Library Association, 1987.

Walter, Virginia A. *Output Measures and More: Planning and Evaluating Public Library Services for Young Adults*. Chicago: American Library Association, 1995.

Walter, Virginia A. *Output Measures for Public Library Services to Children*. Chicago: American Library Association, 1992.

Zweizig, Douglas and others. *The TELL IT! Manual*. Chicago: American Library Association, 1996.

Serving Library Patrons with Disabilities: A Bibliography

Access Board. *Accessible Computer Technology: Meeting the Needs of People with Disabilities.* Tampa, FL: Thompson Publishing Group, 1999.

Alliance for Technology Access. *Computer and Web Resources for People with Disabilities.* 3d. ed. Alameda, CA: Hunter House Publishing, 2000.

Applin, Mary Beth. "Instructional Services for Students with Disabilities." *Journal of Academic Librarianship* 25 (2): 139-142, March 1999.

Balas, Janet L. "Online Resources for Adaptive Information Technologies." *Computers in Libraries* 19(6):38-40, June 1999.

Basu, S. G. *Public Library Services to Visually Disabled Children.* Jefferson, NC: McFarland and Company, 1991.

Beck, Susan Gilbert. "Technology for the Deaf: Remembering to Accommodate an Invisible Disability." *Library Hi Tech* vol. 13, pages 109-122, 1995.

Black, J.B. and others. *Surveying Public Libraries for the ADA.* Tallahassee: State Library of Florida, 1992.

Cirillo, Susan E. and Robert E. Danford. *Library Buildings, Equipment, and the ADA: Compliance Issues and Solutions.* Chicago: ALA, 1996.

Closing the Gap: 2001 Resource Directory. Hutchinson, MN: Closing the Gap, February/March 2001.

"Computer Technology That Can Enable the Disabled." Special issue of *Computers in Libraries* vol. 19, no. 6, June 1999.

Crispen, Joanne, editor. *The Americans With Disabilities Act: Its Impact on Libraries: The Library's Response in Doable Steps.* Chicago: ASCLA/ALA, 1993.

Cunningham, Carmela and Norman Coombs. *Information Access and Adaptive Technology.* Phoenix: Oryx Press, 1997.

Deines-Jones, Courtney and Connie Van Fleet. *Preparing Staff to Serve Patrons with Disabilities: A How-To-Do-It Book.* NY: Neal-Schuman Publishers, 1996.

Dell Orto, Arthur and Robert Marinelli. *Encyclopedia of Disability and Rehabilitation.* NY: MacMillan Library Reference, 1995.
Doerr, D. D. "Compliance: Step-By-Step With the ADA." *Public Library Quarterly* 14(1): 25-29, 1994.

Feinberg, Sandra and others. *Including Families of Children with Special Needs.* NY: Neal-Schuman Publishers, Inc., 1999.

Foos, Donald D. and Nancy C. Pack. *How Libraries Must Comply With the Americans With Disabilities Act.* Phoenix: Oryx Press, 1992.

Friends of Libraries for Deaf Action. *The Red Notebook: Communicating With Hearing People.* National Association of the Deaf. Annual, 1987 - .

Gorman, Audrey. "Libraries Don't Have To Be Confusing Places For Kids With Reading Disabilities." *School Library Journal Online* July 1, 1999.

Gorman, Audrey. "Libraries, Service, and Learning Disabilities." *Knowledge Quest* vol. 27, no.5, p. 20, May/June 1999.

Gorman, Audrey. *Top Twenty LD Resources for Libraries* Chicago: ASCLA/American Library Association, 1999.

Guidelines for Library and Information Services for the American Deaf Community. Chicago: ASCLA/American Library Association, 1996.

Guidelines for Serving People with Mental Retardation. Chicago: ASCLA/American Library Association, 1999.

Gunde, Michael G. "Working with the American with Disabilities Act." *Library Journal* 3 Part Series: December 1991, May 1992, December 1992.

Hagemeyer, Alice. *The Legacy and Leadership of the Deaf Community: A Resource Guide for Librarians and Library Programs.* Chicago: ALA, 1991.

Johnson, David. "Why Is Assistive Technology Underused?" *Library Hi Tech News* #163, June, 1999.

Karp, Rashelle D. *Library Services for Disabled Individuals.* Thorndike, ME: G.K. Hall, 1991.

Klauber, Julie. "An Enabling Collection for People with Disabilities." *Library Journal* v. 121, pages 53-56, April 1996.

Landrum, Judith E. "Adolescent Novels That Feature Characters with Disabilities: An Annotated Bibliography" *Journal of Adolescent and Adult Literacy* 42(4):284-290, December 1998.

LaPlante, Mitchell P. "How Many Americans Have a Disability?" *Disability Statistics Abstract* #5, San Francisco: National Institute on Disability and Rehabilitation Research/US Department of Education, June 1992.

Laurie, Ty D. "Libraries' Duties to Accommodate Their Patrons Under the ADA." *Library Administration and Management* 6(4): 204, Fall 1992.

Lazarro, Joseph. *Adapting PCs for Disabilities*. NY: Addison-Wesley, 1996.

Lazarro, Joseph J. *Adaptive Technologies for Learning and Work Environments*. Chicago: American Library Association, 1993.

Lewis, Christopher. "ADA and its Effect on Libraries." *Public Libraries* 32 (1):24-28, January 1992.

Libraries and the Empowerment of Persons With Disabilities. Special issue of *Library Hi Tech* 14 (1), January 1996

Lilly, Erica B. and Connie Van Fleet. "Wired But Not Connected: Accessibility of Academic Library Pages." *The Reference Librarian* 67/68: 5-28, 1999.

Lisiecki, Christine. "Adaptive Technology for the Library." *Computers in Libraries* 19(6):18-22, June 1999.

Literacy Is For Everyone: Making Library Activities Accessible for Children with Disabilities. Evanston, IL: National Lekotek Center, 1999.

Lovejoy, Eunice. *Portraits of Library Service to People with Disabilities*. Thorndike, ME: G.K. Hall, 1989.

Massachusetts Assistive Technology Partnership. *Assistive Technology: A Basic Training Manual*. Boston: MATP Center, 1999.

Massis, Bruce Edward. *Serving Print Disabled Patrons*. Jefferson, NC: McFarland & Publishers, 1996.

Mates, Barbara T. "Accessible Technology for the '90s: Library Technologies for the Handicapped." *Computers in Libraries*, 13(4):13-16, April 1993.

Mates, Barbara T. *Adaptive Technology for the Internet: Making Electronic Resources Accessible to All*. Chicago: American Library Association, 2000.

Mates, Barbara T. *Library Technology for Visually and Physically Impaired Patrons.* Rev. ed. Westport, CT: Meckler Publishing, 1991.

Mates, Barbara T. "Accessible Technology for the '90s: Library Technologies for the Handicapped." *Computers in Libraries*, 13(4):13-16, April 1993.

Mayo, Kathleen and Ruth O'Donnell, eds. *The ADA Library Kit: Sample ADA-Related Documents to Help You Implement the Law.* Chicago: ASCLA/ALA, 1994.

McNulty, Tom. *Accessible Libraries on Campus: A Practical Guide for the Creation of Disability-Friendly Libraries.* Chicago: Association of College and Research Libraries, 1999.

McNulty, Tom, ed. "Libraries and the Empowerment of People with Disabilities. *Library Hi Tech* vol. 14, pages 23-73, 1996.

McNulty, Tom and Dawn Sorvino. *Access to Information: Materials, Technologies, and Services for Print-Impaired Readers.* LITA Monographs #2. Chicago: American Library Association, 1993.

Miller, Nancy B. and Catherine C. Sammons. *Everybody's Different:* Understanding *and Changing Our Reactions to Disabilities.* Baltimore: Brookes Publishing County., Inc., 1999.

Morgan, Eric L. "Adaptive Technologies for Better Service." *Computers in Libraries* 19(6):35-37, June 1999.

National Council on Disability. *Meeting the Unique Needs of Minorities With Disabilities.* DC: National Council on Disability, 1993.

Norlin, Dennis A. and others. *A Directory of Adaptive Technologies to Aid Library Patrons and Staff With Disabilities.* Chicago: LITA/ALA, 1994.

Norton, Melanie J. And Gail L. Kovalik. "Libraries Serving an Underserved Population: Deaf and Hearing Impaired Patrons." *Library Trends* 41(1): full issue, Summer 1992.

O'Donnell, Ruth and others. "A Core Collection of ADA Information: From the ADA Assembly of ASCLA." *RQ* 33:328-334, Spring 1994.

Pontau, Donna Z. "Transforming Academic Libraries for Employees and Students" in *Diversity and Multiculturalism in Libraries.* Katherine H. Hill, ed. JAI Press, 1994.

Rouse, Veronica. "Making the WEB Accessible." *Computers in Libraries* 19(6): 48-50, June 1999.

Saunders, Laverna. "Removing Obstacles to Provide Equal Access for All Users." *Computers in Libraries* 19(6): 41-47, June 1999.

Schuyler, Michael. "Adapting for Impaired Patrons." *Computers in Libraries* 19(6): 24-29, June 1999.

Switzer, T. R. "The ADA: Creating Positive Awareness and Attitudes." *Library Administration and Management* 8: 205-207, Fall 1994.

Turner, Ray. *Library Patrons With Disabilities.* San Antonio, TX: White Buffalo Press, 1995.

Velleman, Ruth. *Meeting the Needs of People with Disabilities.* Phoenix: Oryx Press, 1990.

Walker, Evelyn, ed. *Programming for Children with Special Needs.* Chicago: American Library Association, 1994.

Walling, Linda Lucas and Marilyn H. Karrenbrock. *Disabilities, Children, and Libraries: Administering Services in Public Libraries and School Media Centers.* Denver, CO: Libraries Unlimited, 1993.

Walling, Linda Lucas and Marilyn M. Irwin. *Information Services for People With Developmental Disabilities: The Library Manager's Handbook.* Westport, CT: Greenwood Press, 1995.

Weingand, Darlene. "The Invisible Client: Meeting the Needs of Persons with Learning Disabilities." *The Reference Librarian* no. 31, pages 77-88, 1990.

Wilhelmus, David W. "Perspectives on the ADA: Accessibility of Academic Libraries to Visually Impaired Patrons." *Journal of Academic Librarianship* 22 (5): 366-370, September 1996.

Wlodkowski, Tom. "Making CD-ROM's Multimedia Work for All Users." *Computers in Libraries* 19(6): 62-66, June 1999.

Wright, Kieth C. And Judith F. Davie. *Serving The Disabled: A How-To-Do-It Manual for Librarians.* NY: Neal-Schuman Publishers, 1991.

Wright, Kieth C. And Judith F. Davie. *Libraries and the Disabled: the Library Manager's Handbook.* Westport, CT: Greenwood Press, 1991.

See also two monthly newsletters on the topic: *FOCUS: Library Service to Older Adults and People With Disabilities.* Edited by Marilyn Irwin and published by the Indiana Institute on Disability and Community, Center for Disability Information and Referral, 2853 E. 10th Street, Bloomington, IN 47408. And *Disabilities Resources Monthly.* Disability Resources, Inc. Four Glatter Lane, Centereach, NY 11720.

Directory of State Offices on Disability

ALABAMA

Governor's Committee on Employment of People with Disabilities
Department of Rehabilitation Service
P.O. Box 11586
Montgomery, AL 36111-0586
(334) 281-8780 (Voice/TTY)
(334) 288-1104 (FAX)

ALASKA

Governor's Committee on Employment and Rehabilitation of People with Disabilities
801 W. 10th Street, Suite A
Juneau, AK 99801-1894
(907) 465-6922 (Voice)
(907) 465-2856 (FAX)
www.labor.state.ak.us/govscomm/index.htm

ARIZONA

Governor's Committee on Employment of People with Disabilities
1012 E. Willetta, SRI-1Bb
Phoenix, AZ 85006
(602) 239-4762 (Voice)
(602) 239-5256 (FAX)

ARKANSAS

Governor's Commission on Employment of People with Disabilities
Arkansas Rehabilitation Services
1616 Brookwood Drive
Little Rock, AR 72202
(501) 296-1626 (Voice/TTY)
(501) 296-1655 (FAX)

CALIFORNIA

California Governor's Committee for Employment of Disabled Persons
EDD, P.O. Box 826880, MIC 41
Sacramento, CA 94280-0001
(916) 654-8055 (Voice)
(916) 654-9820 (TTY)
(916) 654-9821 (FAX)
www.edd.cahwnet.gov/gcedpind.htm

COLORADO

Colorado Governor's Advisory Council for Persons with Disabilities
P.O. Box 15
Golden, CO 80402
(303) 278-9899 (Voice/Fax)
(888) 887-9135 (In State Only)
pw1.netcom.com/~cliffmau/ability.html

CONNECTICUT

Governor's Committee on Employment of People with Disabilities
State of Connecticut Department of Labor
200 Folly Brook Boulevard
Wethersfield, CT 06109
(860) 263-6593 (Voice)
(860) 263-6074 (TTY)
(860) 263-6216 (FAX)

DELAWARE

Governor's Committee on Employment of People with Disabilities
DVR, P.O. Box 9969
Wilmington, DE 19809-0969
(302) 761-8275 (Voice)
(302) 761-6611 (FAX)

DISTRICT OF COLUMBIA

Mayor's Committee on Persons with Disabilities
810 First Street, NE
Room 10015
Washington, DC 20002
(202) 442-8673 (Voice)
(202) 442-8742 (FAX)

FLORIDA

The Able Trust/Florida Governor's Alliance
106 East College Avenue, Suite 820
Tallahassee, FL 32301
(850) 224-4493 (Voice)
(850) 224-4496 (FAX)
www.abletrust.org

GEORGIA

Georgia Committee on Employment of People with Disabilities, Inc.
6810 Creekview Court
Columbus, GA 31904
706-324-2150 (Voice)
706-324-4549 (FAX)

GUAM

Governor's Commission on Persons with Disabilities
Department of Integrated Services for Individuals with Disabilities
1313 Central Avenue
Tiyan, Guam 96913
(671) 475-4698 (Voice)
(671) 477-2892 (FAX)

HAWAII

Disability and Communication Access Board
919 Ala Moana Blvd.
Suite 101
Honolulu, HI 96814
(808) 586-8121 (Voice/TTY)
(808) 586-8129 (FAX)
www.state.hi.us/health/dcab

IDAHO

Governor's Committee on Employment of People with Disabilities
Idaho Department of Labor
317 West Main Street
Boise, ID 83735
(208) 334-6264 (Voice)
(208) 334-6424 (TTY)
(208) 334-6300 (FAX)

ILLINOIS

Office of Rehabilitation Services
James R. Thompson Center
100 West Randolph St., Suite 8-100
Chicago, IL 60601
(312) 814-4036 (Voice)
(312) 814-5000 (TTY)
(312) 814-5849 (FAX)
www.state.il.us/agency/dhs/rsnp.html

INDIANA

Governor's Planning Council for People with Disabilities
143 West Market Street
Indianapolis, IN 46204
(317) 232-7770 (Voice)
(317) 232-7771 (TTY)
(317) 233-3712 (FAX)
http://www.state.in.us/gpcpd

IOWA

Commission of Persons with Disabilities
Department of Human Rights
Lucas State Office Building
321 East 12th Street
Des Moines, IA 50319
(515) 242-6334 (Voice)
(888) 219-0471 (Toll Free)
(515) 242-6119 (FAX)
www.state.ia.us/government/dhr/pd

KANSAS

Kansas Commission on Disability Concerns
1430 S.W. Topeka Blvd.
Topeka, KS 66612-1877
(800) 295-5232 (Toll-free Voice)
(877) 340-5874 (Toll-free TTY)
(785) 296-6525 (Voice)
(785) 296-5044 (TTY)
(785) 296-0466 (FAX)
adabbs.hr.state.ks.us/dc

KENTUCKY

Kentucky Committee on Employment of People with Disabilities
DES Employment Services
275 E. Main Street
2nd Floor West
Frankfort, KY 40621
(502) 564-5331 (Voice/TTY)
(502) 564-7799 (FAX)

LOUISIANA

Governor's Office of Disability Affairs
P.O. Box 94004
Baton Rouge, LA 70804
(225) 219-7547 (Voice)
(225) 219-7550 (Voice/TTY)
(225) 219-7551 (FAX)
(877) 668-2722 (Toll Free)
www.gov.state.la.us/disabilityaffairs/

MAINE

Subcommittee on Disabilities
Creative Work Systems/Maine Jobs Council
443 Congress Street
Portland, ME 04101
(207) 879-1140 (Voice)
(207) 879-1146 (FAX)

MARYLAND

Governor's Committee on Employment of People with Disabilities
Office for Individuals with Disabilities
1 Market Center, Box 10
300 West Lexington Street, 2nd Floor
Baltimore, MD 21201-3435
(410) 333-2263 (Voice/TTY)
(410) 333-6674 (FAX)
www.mdtap.org/oid.html

MASSACHUSETTS

Governor's Commission on Employment of People with Disabilities
Department of Employment and Training
Policy Office
19 Stanford Street, 3rd Floor
Boston, MA 02114
(617) 626-5190 (Voice)
(617) 727-0315 (FAX)

MICHIGAN

Michigan Commission on Disability Concerns
P.O. Box 30659
Lansing, MI 48909
(517) 334-8000 (Voice/TTY)
(517) 334-6637 (FAX)
www.mfia.state.mi.us/mcdc/mcdc.htm

MINNESOTA

Minnesota State Council on Disability
121 E. 7th Place, Suite 107
St. Paul, MN 55101
(651) 296-1743 (Voice)
(651) 296-5935 (FAX)
www.disability.state.mn.us

MISSISSIPPI

Mississippi Department of Rehabilitation Services
P.O. Box 1698
Jackson, MS 39215-1698
(601) 853-5100 (Voice)
(800) 443-1000 (In State Only)
(601) 853-5325 (FAX)
www.mdrs.state.ms.us

MISSOURI

Governor's Council on Disability
P.O. Box 1668
Jefferson City, MO 65102
(573) 751-2600 (Voice/TTY)
(573) 526-4109 (FAX)
www.dolir.state.mo.us/gcd/

MONTANA

Governor's Advisory Council on Disability
State Personnel Division, Dept. of Administration
P.O. Box 200127
Helena, MT 59620-0127
(406) 444-3794 (Voice)
(800) 243-4091 Montana State Relay
(406) 444-0544 (FAX)

NEBRASKA

Governor's Committee on Employment of People with Disabilities
Nebraska Workforce Development, Department of Labor
P.O. Box 94600
Lincoln, NE 68509-4600
(402) 471-3405 (Voice)
(402) 471-2318 (FAX)

NEVADA

Governor's Committee on Employment of People with Disabilities
4600 Kietzke Lane
Suite A108
Reno, NV 89502
(775) 688-1111 (Voice/TTY)
(775) 688-1113 (FAX)

NEW HAMPSHIRE

Governor's Commission on Disability
57 Regional Drive
Concord, NH 03301-8518
(603) 271-2773 (Voice/TTY)
(603) 271-2837 (FAX)
(800) 852-3405 (Toll Free)
webster.state.nh.us/disability/

NEW JERSEY

New Jersey Department of Labor
P.O. Box 398
Trenton, NJ 08625-0398
(609) 292-7959 (Voice)
(609) 292-8347 (FAX)
www.state.nj.us/labor/dvrs/dvr.html

NEW MEXICO

Governor's Committee on Concerns of the Handicapped
Lamy Building - Room 117
491 Old Santa Fe Trail
Santa Fe, NM 87501
(505) 827-6465 (Voice)
(505) 827-6329 (TTY)
(505) 827-6328 (FAX)
www.state.nm.us/gcch/gcch.htm

NEW YORK

New York State Office of Advocate for Persons with Disabilities
One Empire State Plaza, Suite 1001
Albany, NY 12223-1150
(518) 473-4129 (Voice)
(800) 522-4369 (In State Only)
(518) 473-4231 (TTY)
(518) 473-6005 (FAX)
www.advoc4disabled.state.ny.us/

NORTH CAROLINA

The North Carolina Employment Network
2801 Mail Service Center
Raleigh, NC 27699-2801
(919) 733-3364 (Voice)
(919) 733-7968 (FAX)

NORTH DAKOTA

Governor's Committee on Employment of People with Disabilities
600 South 2nd Street, Suite 1B
Bismarck, ND 58504
(701) 328-8952 (Voice)
(701) 328-8969 (FAX)

OHIO

Ohio Governor's Council on People with Disabilities
400 East Campus View Boulevard
Columbus, OH 43235-4604
(614) 438-1393 (Voice)
(614) 438-1274 (FAX)
(800) 282-4536 Ext. 1391 (In State Only)
www.state.oh.us/gcpd/

OKLAHOMA

Governor's Committee on Employment of People with Disabilities
Shepherd Mall
2712 Villa Prom
Oklahoma City, OK 73107-2423
(405) 521-3756 (Voice/TTY)
(405) 522-6695 (FAX)
www.state.ok.us/~ohc

OREGON

Oregon Disabilities Commission
1257 Ferry Street S.E.
Salem, OR 97310
(503) 378-3142 (Voice/TTY)
(503) 378-3599 (FAX)
www.odc.state.or.us

PENNSYLVANIA

Governor's Committee on Employment of People with Disabilities
909 Green Street
Harrisburg, PA 17102
(717) 783-5231 (Voice)
(717) 783-5221 (FAX)

PUERTO RICO

Governor's Committee on Employment of People with Disabilities
Office of the Ombudsman for Persons with Disabilities
P.O. Box 41309
San Juan, PR 00940-1309
(787) 725-2333 ext. 2070 (Voice)
(787) 725-4014 (TTY)
(787) 721-2455 (FAX)
www.oppi.prstar.net

RHODE ISLAND

Governor's Commission on Disabilities
Howard Complex
41 Cherry Dale Court
Cranston, RI 02920-3049
(401) 462-0100 (Voice)
(401) 462-0101 (TTY)
(401) 462-0106 (FAX)
www.gcd.state.ri.us

SOUTH CAROLINA

Governor's Committee on Employment of People with Disabilities
South Carolina Vocational Rehabilitation Department
P.O. Box 15
West Columbia, SC 29171-0015
(803) 896-6580 (Voice)
(803) 896-6510 (FAX)

SOUTH DAKOTA

Board of Vocational Rehabilitation
221 South Central Avenue
Pierre, SD 57501
(605) 945-2207 (Voice)
(605) 945-2422 (FAX)
www.state.sd.us/dhs/drs/

TENNESSEE

Tennessee Committee for Employment of People with Disabilities
Division of Rehabilitation Services
Citizens Plaza Building, Room 1100
400 Deaderick Street
Nashville, TN 37248-6000
(615) 313-4891 (Voice)
(615) 313-5695 (TTY)
(615) 741-6508 (FAX)

TEXAS

Governor's Committee on People with Disabilities
Governor's Office
P.O. Box 12428
Austin, TX 78711
(512) 463-5742 (Voice)
(512) 463-5746 (TTY)
(512) 463-5745 (FAX)
www.governor.state.tx.us/disabilities

UTAH

Utah Governor's Committee on Employment of People with Disabilities
1595 West 500 South
Salt Lake City, UT 84104
(801) 887-9529 (Voice)
(801) 278-9844 (FAX)

VERMONT

The Governor's Committee on Employment of People with Disabilities
1187 Maple Street
Waterbury Center, VT 05677
(802) 241-2612 (Voice/DDC)
(802) 244-5075 (FAX)
www.hireus.org

VIRGINIA

Virginia Board for People with Disabilities
202 North 9th Street
9th Floor
Richmond VA 23219
(804) 786-0016(Voice/TTY)
(800) 846-4464 (Voice/TTY) (In State Only)
(804) 786-1118 (FAX)
www.vaboard.org/

VIRGIN ISLANDS

Division of Disabilities and Vocational Rehabilitation Services
Department of Human Services
Knud Hansen Complex - Building A
1303 Hospital Ground
St. Thomas, Virgin Islands 00802-4355
(340) 774-2323 Ext. 2134 (Voice)
(340) 773-3641 (FAX)

WASHINGTON

Governor's Committee on Disability Issues and Employment
P.O. Box 9046
Olympia, WA 98507-9046
(360) 438-3168 (Voice)
(360) 438-3167 (TTY)
(360) 438-3208 (FAX)

WEST VIRGINIA

Division of Rehabilitation Services
State Capitol Complex
P.O. Box 50890
Charleston, WV 25305-0890
(304) 766-4601 (Voice)
(304) 766-4965 (TTY)
(304) 766-4905 (FAX)
www.wvdrs.org

WISCONSIN

Governor's Committee for People with Disabilities
P.O. Box 7850
Madison, WI 53707-7851
(608) 267-4896 (Voice)
(608) 267-7376 (TTY)
(608) 264-9832 (FAX)

WYOMING

Governor's Committee on Employment of People with Disabilities
1st Floor - East Wing
Herschler Building, Room 1126
Cheyenne, WY 82002
(307) 777-7191 (Voice/TTY)
(307) 777-5939 (FAX)
wydoe.state.wy.us/doe.asp?ID=122

Internet Resources for Disability and Accessibility Information

ABLEDATA www.abledata.com

Accessible Web Page Design: Resources
http://library.uwsp.edu/aschmetz/accessible/pub_resources.htm#legal_
info

ADA and Disability Information
www.public.iastate.edu/~sbilling/ada.html

Alliance for Technology Access http://www.ataccess.org

American with Disabilities Act Information
www.usdoj.gov/crt/ada/ada-home.html

American Foundation for the Blind (AFB): www.igc.apc.org/afb/

American Speech-Language-Hearing Association: www.asha.org

Assistive Technology Issues: www.tsbvi.edu/technology/

Blindness Resource Center: www.nyise.org/blind.htm

Center for Applied Special Technology: www.cast.org

Center on Information Technology Accommodation (CITA):
    www.itpolicy.gsa.gov/coca/index.html

Closing the Gap: www.closingthegap.com

Deaf Resource Library: www.deaflibrary.org/

Deaf World Web: www.deafworldweb.org

Disability and Business Technical Assistance Center (for New England): www.adaptenv.org

>   *Note:* Offers technical assistance to libraries too. For human help, call 617-695-1225 or E-mail at adaptive@adaptenv.org

Disability Law: www.law.cornell.edu/topics/disability.html or www.ferleger.com/

Disability Resource List: www.eskimo.com/~jlubin/disabled.html

Disability Resources Webwatcher: www.disabilityresources.org/DRMwww.html

Disability Resources Regional Resource Directory www.disabilityresources.org/DRMreg.html

Disability Statistics Center: http://128.218.183.95/ucsf/spl.taf

DO-IT (Disabilities, Opportunities,Internetworking & Technology) www:washington.edu/doit

Easy Access to Software and Information (EASI): www.rit/edu/~easi

LD Online (Learning Disabilities): www.ldonline.org

Library Web Pages Which Comply with the ADA www.librarylaw.com/ADAwebpage.html

Meta Index to Disability Resources on the Web: www.gen.emory.edu/medweb/medweb.disabled.html

Mental Health Internet: www.mirconnect.com/national/index.html

National Center for Health Statistics: www.cdc.gov/nchswww
Note: For human help, call 301-436-8500.

National Center for Information on Deafness (Gallaudet): www.gallaudet.udu

National Council on Disability: www.ncd.gov

National Information Center for Children and Youth with Disabilities: www.nichcy.org

National Institute of Mental Health: www.nimh.nih.gov
    Note: For human help, call 301-443-4513 or E-mail to nimhinfo@nih.gov

National Institute on Deafness and Other Communications Disorders:
    www.nih.gov/nicd

National Institute on Disability and Rehabilitation Research:
    www.dsc.ucsf.edu/ or www.infouse.com/disabilitydata/

National Library Service for the Blind & Physically Handicapped:
    www.loc.goc/nls/

National Organization on Disability: www.nod.org
    Note: For human help, call 202-293-5960.

National Rehabilitation Information Center (NARIC) Instant Disability Information Center: www.naric.com/search/

Statistics on Children with Visual Impairments:
    www.lighthouse.org/educ_stats1.htm

Trace Research and Development Center: www.trace.wisc.edu/

US Census Bureau   www.census.gov/
    Note: From Web page, select "Subjects A-Z" and click on "D." Then choose "Disability," and then "Americans with Disabilities: 1994-95." For human help, call 301-457-3242 or E-mail to hhes-info@census.gov.

Women and Disability in the US: www.nces.ed.gov/pubs99/1999187.pdf

World Institute on Disability: wid.com

Federal Disability Data Resources

Who are people with disabilities? What do we know about people with disabilities? How many individuals with disabilities use assistive devices? How many people with disabilities are working? What are people with disabilities' demographics? These are just a few of the questions that are asked every day as we develop and implement programs and strategies to combat the high unemployment rate of persons with disabilities. Numerous resources are available to provide statistical data to answer these questions and provide information on other disability related topics. Many resources now post their information on Web sites which makes researching disability data readily accessible and fast. Outlined below is information on some of the data resources regarding people with disabilities.

National Center on Health Statistics (NCHS)

The National Center on Health Statistics in 1998 made available national information on assistive devices used by people with disabilities from their National Health Interview Survey on Disability (NHIS-D), conducted in 1994. This is the first time national data on the use of assistive devices by people with disabilities has ever been released. The data covers: anatomical devices (braces, artificial limbs), mobility devices, hearing devices and vision devices. The complete NHIS-D survey is available in NCHS's Web site: www.cdc.gov/nchswww/default.htm~http://www.cdc.gov/nchswww/default.htm. To obtain a print or CD-ROM copy, call (301) 436-7551. A CD-ROM is also available which offers far more disability data than appears either on their Web site or is available in print.

National Organization on Disability (NOD)

The 1998 National Organization on Disability/Harris Poll of Americans with Disabilities, a nationwide survey of 1,000 Americans with disabilities aged 16 and older, was conducted in mid-1998. This survey found that Americans with disabilities continue to lag well behind other Americans in many of the most basic aspects of life. Large gaps still exist between adults with disabilities and other adults with regard to employment, education, income, frequency of socializing and other basic measures of ten major "indicator" areas of life. Furthermore, most of these gaps show little evidence of narrowing. In some cases, the gaps have even widened over time.

Employment continues to be the area with the widest gulf between those who are disabled and those who are not. Forty two percent of those who are disabled and not working believe that attitudinal barriers keep them from working (i.e., that employers are unwilling to recognize that they are capable of taking on a full-time job). A significant majority of people with disabilities who work (64 percent) and people with disabilities who want to work (81 percent) have encountered supervisors and co-workers who are afraid that a person with a disability "cannot do the job."

The study provided some interesting data on the use of technology by persons with disabilities.

- Only one in four (25 percent) of individuals with disabilities who work and four out of ten (40 percent) of individuals with disabilities who want to work say they need special equipment or technology to perform effectively the kind of job they prefer.

- Half (49 percent) of people with disabilities who work full or part-time use computers at work. Those who work full-time are much more likely (60 percent) to use a computer than those who work part-time (35 percent).

- More than a quarter (28 percent) of people with disabilities own special equipment or technology to assist them because of their disability. The number has risen significantly since 1994 when it was 22 percent. Those who describe their disability as very or somewhat severe are more likely (33 percent) to own special equipment than those who characterize their disability as slight or moderate (19 percent).

- Fifteen percent of people with disabilities who work full or part-time, or would like to be working, need a personal computer.

For more information on this study visit NOD's Web site:

www.nod.org, or call (202) 283-5960 (V) or (202) 293-5968 (TDD).

The National Institute on Disability and Rehabilitation Research (NIDRR)

The National Institute on Disability and Rehabilitation Research is a federal government agency charged with maintaining disability statistics. Recently, NIDRR published "Chartbook on Work and Disability in the United States, 1998," a compendium of key findings from numerous statistical sources. It can be viewed on the Web site, or in print copy.

Web site: www.disabilitydata.com~http://www.disabilitydata.com
Phone: (202) 205-5633 (V)

Disability Statistics Center

The Disability Statistics Center is a national center of research and training. The Center receives its primary funding from NIDRR. The Center has ongoing research projects on the cost of disability, employment and earnings, access to health and long-term care services, housing, mortality and national statistical indicators on the status of people with disabilities in America.

Web site: www.dsc.ucsf.edu/~http://www.dsc.ucsf.edu/
Phone: (415)502-5217 (V)

The Census Bureau

The Census Bureau plans to include questions on disability in the 2000 Census. In the meantime, the Census Bureau maintains a disability statistics Web site. The statistics include information on the numbers of persons with disabilities on a state-by-state and metropolitan area basis.

Web site: www.census.gov/hhes/www/disability.html
Phone: (301) 457-3242 (V)

Disability Statistics and Terminology

Terminology

The basic current American definition of *disability* assumes activity limitation due to mental or physical impairment or chronic disease. (The World Health Organization still uses the term "handicapped" which is considered derogatory in the US). An *impairment* refers to how a body is structured or how it functions. A person with a disability either cannot perform, or finds it difficult to perform, a major life activity. Note that impairment and disability are not the same, as some impairments do not interfere with life activities and so are not considered disabling. *Functional limitation* is similar to *disability* except that it focuses on incapacity and difficulty in doing actions rather than activities. *Actions* are defined as physical or mental interactions with the world, such as talking, thinking, and walking. *Activities* are complex groupings of actions such as working, playing or reading a newspaper. (1)

Another broad term used in the field is *work disability* The Census defines it as a limitation in a person's ability to work due to a physical, mental, or other health condition that has lasted at least six months. Severe work disability means a person is prevented from working at a job while nonsevere work disability means the person is limited in the kind or amount of work. According to the National Institute on Disability and Rehabilitation Research, in Massachusetts, 36.3% of people with a work disability are working.

Each disability has more than one name, depending on what agency or organization is using it and depending on the political bent of the user. "Mental illness" is a term used by medical and mental health professionals for serious impairments of thought and feeling. "Mental disorder" means the same thing but is currently used by non-medical professionals to avoid the word "illness" with its medical model connotations. Similarly, the deaf community uses "late-deafened" for people who lose their hearing after acquiring language fluency and usually do not primarily define themselves as deaf and do not use sign language (ASL). "Deaf" people – with a capital D – consider themselves a cultural group with their own distinct language (ASL). Most Deaf people were born deaf.

And disabilities are grouped in varying ways as well. For example, the National Center for Health Statistics has a category "mental disability" which covers "mental retardation, Alzheimer's disease, senility, dementia, learning disabilities, or any other mental or emotional condition." Note that this category includes three groups of conditions which are usually kept separate: mental retardation which is ordinarily considered a developmental disability, mental disorders, and learning disabilities. Another example is that "sensory disorders" includes impairments of all five senses while "communication disorders" covers deaf and hard of hearing people and people with speech disorders. Clearly deaf and hard of hearing people are included in both groups so such categories cannot be easily compared.

Statistics

In the ADA legislation, 43 million Americans – or 20% of the population – were cited as having disabilities. This number, however, is often contested. According to Mitchell L. LaPlante, a major researcher in the field of disability statistics, the 43 million people included people with any impairment, minimal to severe, yet did not include people with activity limitations due to chronic disease. (2)

Every other statistic offered for the number of Americans with disabilities is equally vulnerable to criticism. There is no one "correct answer." Each year, agencies of the US government compile and publish statistics relating to disability. However, these statistics – as well as the definition of the term "disability" and the age categories used – are not standardized, making it nearly impossible to find one accurate number or even several comparable numbers.

One blatant example is that the National Center for Health Statistics and Gallaudet University state that 8.6% of people have hearing impairments while the US National Health Survey number is 1.9%. The larger number (which is used as the standard and was adopted by most states) includes deafness while the 1.9% does not.

The three most significant sources for government information on disabilities are the National Health Information Survey (NHIS), the Current Population Survey (CPS), and the Survey on Income and Program Participation (SIPP). All are collected by the US Census but each has a separate sponsor which is looking for its own data. The NHIS is sponsored by the National Center for Health Statistics, the CPS is sponsored by the US Bureau of Labor Statistics, and the SIPP is sponsored by the Census. All of the collected data are regarded as "estimates" because of sampling and non-sampling errors.

A fourth often quoted source is the National Medical Expenditure Survey (NMES), a 1987 study by the Agency for Health Care Policy and Research of the US Department of Health and Human Services.

A brief overview of how these four collect and categorize their data demonstrates how difficult it is to compare information among them or to find one "correct" statistic.

The NHIS is a large annual national survey of a sample of non-institutionalized people who are interviewed as to whether they are limited in the major activities in their particular age group or are limited in other areas (non-major) because of a physical or mental impairment existing or expected to last for at least three months. The NHIS uses the following categories: children 5-17 for whom the major activity is attending school, adults 18-69 for whom the major activity is working or keeping house, and people 70 and over whose major activity is independent living. According to the NHIS, the three most prevalent disabling conditions are orthopedic impairments, arthritis, and heart disease.
The 1990 NHIS estimated that 22.9 million people of all ages living in households are limited in major activity. An additional 10.9 million people have "non-major" activity limitations. This totals to 33.8 million or 13.7% of the US population not residing in institutions who have some activity limitations. When census data on institutional residents with activity limitations are added in, the total comes to 36.1 million people or 14.5%. The NHIS estimates are the most commonly used but are lower than some others. (3)

The CPS is a monthly survey of approximately 50,000 households. It is the primary source of information on US labor force characteristics in the civilian non-institutionalized population. Households are asked about the employment status of each member of the household fifteen years of age and over. In asking about employment it uncovers information on work disabilities. It uses the following age categories: 16-18, 19-64, and 65+.

The SIPP is a monthly survey of 8,000 living units. It gathers information on the income sources of non-institutionalized people in the US. As part of this, it collects information on people with functional (rather than activity) limitations due to physical or sensory impairments. Unlike the NHIS which asks about a specific activity it has established as important for the age group (e.g. working), the SIPP asks about actions such as getting around inside and outside the home, speaking, listening, seeing, ascending stairs, lifting sixty pounds, and walking a quarter mile. The SIPP age categories are 3-5, 6-14, 15-24, 25-34, 35-44, 45-54, 55-64, 65-74, and 75+.

The NMES was a national survey of a sample of the civilian population including non-institutionalized people and persons living in nursing homes and facilities for people with mental retardation. People were asked about their difficulties in performing basic life activities dues to mental or physical health problems. They reported two categories of activities. The first was self-care, called "activities of daily living" (ADL), such as bathing, dressing, toileting, feeding oneself and getting about the home. The other were community and home management activities, called "instrumental activities of daily living" (IADL), such as household chores, handling money, shopping, and getting about the community (outside the home). Difficulty in ADL and IADL was measured by the nature and amount of assistance necessary. The age-breakdowns for the NMES were 0-17, 18-44, 45-54, 55-64, 65-74, 75-84, and 85+. The NMES was last done in 1987. Now named the Medical Expenditure Survey (MEPS), it became linked to the NHIS in 1996 and now shares its data.

K-12 school districts also collect, compile, and publish statistics. These only include children who are enrolled in school. The data is organized by grade and/or school level. The IDEA requires them to keep figures for 12 disability categories: specific learning disabilities, hearing impairments, speech or language impairments, visual impairments, autism, deaf-blindness, traumatic brain injury, multiple disabilities, other health impairments, mental retardation, serious emotional disturbance, and orthopedic impairments. Community college, colleges, and universities keep data which is reported to the National Center for Education Statistics at the US Department of Education. This information is kept by undergraduate and graduate in six disability categories: visual impairment, hearing impairment or deaf, speech impairment, orthopedic impairment, learning disability, other disability or impairment.

In the scan forms and the glossary for this process, statistics are given as formulas for extrapolating local statistics. The statistics given may have derived from one of the national surveys, but have also been corroborated by an organization or agency focused on the specific disability. Using statistics that are locally gathered and analyzed is the safest way to determine who is in your community.

Notes

1) La Plante, Mitchell P. "Who Counts as Having a Disability? Musings on the Meanings and Prevalence of Disability." *Disabilities Studies Quarterly* 10 (3): 15-17, 1990.

2) La Plante, Mitchell P. "How Many Americans Have a Disability?" *Disability Statistics Abstract #5*. SF: National Institute on Disability and Rehabilitation Research, June 1992.

3) Dell Orto, Arthur and Robert Marinelli. *Encyclopedia of Disability and Rehabilitation.* NY: MacMillan Library Reference, 1995.

What to Say: Language About Disabilities

Accepted terminology about disabilities changes regularly. From derogatory expressions to medical terms, from euphemisms to politically crafted phrases, the words used to describe people with disabilities have evolved to reflect a growing awareness of disabilities and positive attitudes towards all sorts of people.

Three basic guidelines for language about disabilities:

The primary rule is to put ***people first***. In other words, emphasize the ***person***, not the disability. For example, instead of describing people as "disabled customers," call them "customers with disabilities." Similarly, don't refer to people as their disability. Say "People with developmental disabilities" rather than "The developmentally disabled." Say "He had epilepsy" instead of "He was epileptic."

Secondly, stress the ***ability***, not the disability. So instead of saying "Although she has cerebral palsy, Juan manages to write a weekly newspaper column," note that "Juan writes a weekly newspaper column." If necessary to the context, add "He has cerebral palsy."

Last, underline the ***positive***, not the negative. For example, instead of portraying Susan as a "victim of polio," say "Susan survived polio" or "Susan lives with polio." Another example is to substitute "Kareem uses a wheelchair" for "Kareem is wheelchair-bound."

Don't Use:	*Do Use:*
abnormal	person with a disability
afflicted with	person with …
cerebral-palsied	person with cerebral palsy
confined to a wheelchair	wheelchair user
crazy	person who is mentally ill
crippled, crip	person with a motor disability or orthopedic impairment

Don't Use:	**Do Use:**
deaf and dumb	person with hearing & speech impairments or language impairments or multiple disabilities
deaf mute	person with hearing/speech impairments or language impairments multiple disabilities
defective	person with a disability
deformed	person with a disability
deinstitutionalized	person who no longer lives in an institution
dumb, mute	person who is unable to speak or uses synthetic speech
epileptic	person with epilepsy
fit	seizure
gimp	person with a disability
handicapped	person with a disability
insane	person with a mental illness
invalid	person with a disability
lame	person with a motor disability or with a mobility impairment
maimed	person with a disability
normal	person without disabilities or who is able-bodied
paralytic	person with a motor disability or who is paralyzed
restricted to a wheelchair	wheelchair user or person in a wheelchair
retard	person who is developmentally disabled or who has mentally retardation
spastic or spaz	person with cerebral palsy or person who has seizures
stricken	person with ...
stutterer	person with a speech impairment
sufferer	person with ...
survivor	person living with ...
the blind	people who are blind
the deaf	people who are deaf
the disabled	people with disabilities
victim	person with ...
wheelchair-bound	wheelchair user or person in a wheelchair

Do not avoid using typical expressions that refer to the senses such as "See you later," "It's good to see you," or "Got to run."

Tip Sheets for Communicating with People with Disabilities

Serving Patrons Who Are Deaf or Hard of Hearing

People who are <u>deaf</u> are unable to rely on audition alone to understand speech; they must also rely on visual and other cues. People who are <u>hard of hearing</u> have difficulty hearing speech without amplification. There are many techniques and accommodations which can help hearing people communicate with people who are deaf or hard of hearing. Communication modes with deaf and hard of hearing patrons will vary depending on residual hearing, age of onset of hearing loss, speechreading or sign language skills, and personal preferences.

Communication Methods

- **American Sign Language (ASL).** A visual based language with its own grammar and syntax, ASL is the primary language of the deaf community in the United States. (Most hard of hearing adults, however, rely on assistive listening devices such as hearing aids and telephone amplifiers.) ASL interpreters facilitate communication between deaf and hearing individuals by conveying spoken English in ASL and vice versa.
- **Written English.** Deaf and hard of hearing people may communicate with hearing people by reading and writing English. In one-to-one interactions in the library this may mean simply writing notes back and forth with paper and pen or on a nearby computer. Note that many deaf people, especially those who have never heard English, have difficulty mastering English which is a foreign language to them; reading levels may be low so keep written communication simple until you know the abilities of the individual person.
- **Communication Access Realtime Translation (CART).** Another type of interpretation, CART provides visual text with nearly instantaneous translation of the spoken word. The CART provider types the speaker's words on a stenographic machine which is connected to a computer with software to translate the stenographic code into English. The translation can then be read on the computer screen; for larger group events the CART text can be displayed on a large video screen or projected onto the wall.

- **Telecommunications**. **TTY**s, which are sometimes called TDDs or text telephones, are small typewriter-like devices that transmit text over the telephone lines. TV programs and videos are now often captioned (closed captioned require decoding, open captions are visible at all times) for deaf people to read; recent FCC regulations require one hundred percent **captioning** in network and cable broadcasting. Another telecommunications method is the **relay services** mandated by Title IV of the ADA. TTY users can connect to the library via the relay service whose operators will read the text aloud to the hearing staff person who can then respond to the operator who will transmit the return message via TTY.
- **Spoken English**. People who are hard of hearing may be able to communicate orally if an amplification device is used. Deaf people also may communicate orally depending on their training and may be able to "speech read" (previously known as lip reading) if you enunciate clearly.

Tips for Serving Patrons Who are Deaf or Hard of Hearing

- Approach the patron so you can be seen.
- Get the patron's attention before you start speaking.
- Ask the patron how s/he prefers to communicate and then accommodate the request. Do not assume a knowledge of sign language. Do not leave to find a person who can sign unless the patron requests it.
- Reduce background noise or move to a quieter location.
- Always face the patron as you speak and maintain eye contact.
- If you are using an interpreter, be sure to speak directly to the patron, not to the interpreter.
- Speak at a normal pace, enunciating carefully; do not exaggerate your lip movements or mumble as this makes speechreading difficult.
- Keep your mouth visible – do not obscure it with your hands or by chewing gum or food.
- Be aware of the lighting. For example, do not stand in front of a light source because that makes it difficult to speechread or to pick up visual cues.
- If a hard of hearing patron has hearing aids or other assistive listening devices, give her/him an opportunity to adjust the equipment.
- If the patron does not seem to understand you, write it down.

Serving Patrons Who Are Blind or Visually Impaired

People who are *blind* do not see well enough to read (depending on the cause and severity of the blindness, they may, however, see shapes or patterns of light and dark). People who are *visually impaired* may see with correction (glasses, contact lenses, or surgery) or may have severe disabilities which make reading difficult. There are many techniques and accommodations which can assist people who are blind or visually impaired people in using library materials.

Communication Methods

♦ **Voice**. Many blind people have volunteer or paid **readers** who read written materials aloud to them at home, at work, or in the library. **Reading machines** scan printed materials and translate it into speech which is read aloud by a synthesized voice. This technology also allows computers to "talk" so that information on computer (e.g. your library's online catalog) or on CD-ROM can be read (that is, heard) by people who are blind or visually limited. **Descriptive videos** (DVS) allow people who are blind or visually impaired to hear a description of what others are seeing; a narrator describes key visual elements during pauses in the video's regular dialogue.

♦ **Braille**. This is a tactile reading and writing system, created in 1829, consisting of raised dots produced in a six-dot configuration which stand for the letters of the alphabet and certain letter combinations or word contractions. Note that some people who are blind and most people who are visually impaired, especially those who lost vision later in life, do not read Braille. For those who do read Braille, however, it is usually the preferred mode of reading because of its portability and its non-reliance on electronics. Braille can be produced manually, on special typewriters, and on computers with Braille translation software. Some Braille users carry pocket sized Braille computers with them for taking notes; the data can then be read aloud or printed in Braille. The reading machines mentioned above can also produce Braille copy if the proper accessories are attached.

♦ **Magnification**. Many people with limited vision can read large type books and printed materials. (This includes large print key caps on keyboards.) If the materials are in standard print or handwriting-- or if the large type is not large enough – magnification devices can be used. These include hand held magnifiers; closed circuit televisions (**CCTV**s) or electronic magnifiers; screen enlargers which passively magnify a computer's screen; and magnification software which enlarges the print on the computer screen.

Tips for Serving Patrons who are Blind or Visually Impaired

- Do not yell or speak loudly to people with vision loss; most are not deaf or hard of hearing.
- Identify yourself and others with you. If in a group setting remember to identify the person you are addressing.
- Have your voice show your welcome and helpfulness
- Speak directly to the patron, not through her/his sighted companion.
- Do not touch or pet a guide dog on duty.
- When giving directions, use the clock face as your basis. For example, "The reference desk is at 3:00 from where you're facing."
- When guiding a patron, allow the person to take your elbow; do not grab the patron's arm or hand. Stand next to him/her and slightly ahead, then ask her/him to take your arm.
- Ask what you can do to help and which materials format/communication method is preferred.

Serving Patrons with Mobility or Orthopedic Impairments

People with mobility impairments may use canes and/or crutches, walkers, motorized scooters, or wheelchairs to get around. Many of these people are capable of all tasks but walking. Depending on the cause of the disability, other (or additional) voluntary muscles may be affected. For example, a person with a disability may not be able to hold a book or turn pages. Spinal cord injuries, musculoskeletal disorders such as arthritis, and some developmental disabilities such as cerebral palsy are common causes of motor impairments.

Besides personal auxiliary mobility aids such as wheelchairs and canes, other aids for people with motor impairments include wheeled carts for carrying library materials, rolling stools, step stools, reaching devices, book holders, and page turners. Your library may have these for people to use in your facility.

Tips for Serving Patrons With Motor Impairments

✔ Keep clear pathways for people using wheelchairs and canes.
✔ A wheelchair (or scooter or walker) is part of the personal body space of its user. Do not touch it (or push it) without permission.
✔ Do not carry a patron unless it is an emergency evacuation situation or the person requests it.
✔ Place yourself at the patron's eye level by sitting or crouching.
✔ Speak directly to the patron rather than through his/her attendant.
✔ Do not assume speech or other disabilities.
✔ Do not assume they need information on disabilities.
✔ A person using a wheelchair is not "wheelchair bound," "crippled," or "handicapped."
✔ Ask the person how you can help.

Serving Patrons with Learning Disabilities

Learning disabilities – also called learning differences – are neurological disorders that make it difficult for individuals to process and/or interpret sensory information. The disability may manifest itself in only one area (e.g. reading or math) or in many. People with learning disabilities have average or above average intelligence and, with accommodations, can learn at age appropriate levels. Dyslexia and attention deficit disorder (ADD) are the most common examples of learning disabilities, but over 100 different specific learning disabilities have been identified.

Tips for Serving Patrons With Learning Disabilities

- Give clear directions, checking for comprehension, and paraphrasing or repeating if necessary.
- Be patient. A person with a learning disability may need extra time to understand you or to complete a task.
- Be literal. Some people with learning differences have difficulty with tonal subtleties and with metaphors.
- If a form (e.g. library card application) needs completion, offer assistance if writing is a problem.
- Offer information in a variety of reading and comprehension levels and in non-print formats.
- Treat the person with respect. Often people with learning differences are treated as stupid, lazy, or developmentally disabled.

Serving Patrons with Speech Disorders

Speech, voice, and language disorders affect a person's ability to speak in an understandable fashion. There are many causes of speech disorders including cerebral palsy, head injuries, deafness, Parkinson's disease and stroke. People with speech difficulties are of average or above average intelligence, and usually process information without difficulty; the problem lies in communicating with others.

Tips for Serving Patrons with Speech Disorders

- If you are unsure what the person is saying, repeat it back, asking for confirmation that you have understood.
- If you definitely do not understand what the patron is saying, tell him/her and ask how the two of you can communicate more easily.
- Offer writing as an alternative means of communication. Note that some causes of speech difficulty also make writing arduous.
- Consider moving to a quiet, less public area. Stressful situations often exacerbate a person's speech difficulties.
- Be patient. A person with a speech difficulty may need extra time to communicate clearly.
- Do not finish the person's sentences for him/her. This is insulting.
- Treat the person with respect. Often a person with a speech difficulty is treated as drunk, developmentally disabled, or mentally ill.

FOR PHOTOCOPYING

The following pages provide templates of the scans and the budget-planning form found elsewhere in this book, free of running heads and page numbers. You may photocopy them for your use.

LIBRARY SCAN: PLANNING FOR
LIBRARY SERVICES FOR PEOPLE WITH DISABILITIES

1. Does your library comply with the ADA regarding physical accessibility to and within the library facility? Mark Y for yes and N for no.

- _____ Parking spaces
- _____ Ramps and curb cuts
- _____ Building and interior entrances (doors)
- _____ Stairs, floors, and elevators
- _____ Stack aisles
- _____ Reading/ study area aisles and seating areas
- _____ Service counters
- _____ Desks and other furniture
- _____ Telephones
- _____ Drinking fountains
- _____ Alarm systems
- _____ **Signage**
- _____ Bathrooms

2. Does your library have a plan to come into compliance with the ADA by fixing those items marked N?

3. Who is your library's ADA Coordinator?

4. Does your library have an advisory group of people with disabilities?

5. Does your library have any staff members with disabilities? If so, what disabilities?

6. Does your library offer staff ongoing training in the following areas? Mark Y for yes and N for no.

_____ Sensitivity training on disabilities?
_____ Customer service for people with disabilities?
_____ How to be a sighted guide for blind patrons?
_____ Sign language basics?
_____ Local agencies and organizations to whom you can refer people with
      disabilities?
_____ Awareness of special equipment and its availability? (assistive
      technologies)?
_____ How to use the equipment and to assist others in using it?
_____ Federal and state laws concerning services to people with
      disabilities?

7. *What alternative format materials does your library own? Check all that the*
library has.

     _____ Large print books
     _____ Audio books/ books on tape (commercial)
     _____ Talking books (NLS)
     _____ Braille books
     _____ Print/ braille books
     _____ Closed caption videos
     _____ Described videos
     _____ Instructional videos on sign language
     _____ Toys and other tangibles
     _____ Adaptive technology for loan
     _____ Other (please specify)

8. *What special services are offered to patrons with disabilities? Check all that*
are offered.

     _____ Extended loan periods
     _____ Extended reserve periods
     _____ Library cards for caregivers/ proxies
     _____ Ability to check out more than the usual number of materials
     _____ Dial-in access to the OPAC
     _____ Electronic access to library resources from home (or dorm)
     _____ Home delivery service
     _____ Books-by-mail
     _____ Brochures and library maps in alternative formats
     _____ TTY reference service
     _____ Fax access to reference and/or circulation desk
     _____ Email access to reference and/or circulation desk
     _____ ASL or realtime captioning offered at public programs
     _____ Volunteer reader in library

_____ Volunteer technology assistant in library
_____ Radio reading service or Newsline for the Blind
_____ Other (please specify)

9. *What assistive technology (non-computer) does the library offer? Check all the library has.*

_____ Public use TTY/ TTY payphone
_____ Assistive listening devices for use in the library
_____ Assistive listening system in meeting rooms/auditoriums
_____ Hand-held magnifiers for in-library use
_____ Electronic magnifiers (CCTV)
_____ Reacher/ grabbers
_____ Wheelchairs/ scooters for in-house use
_____ Talking signage
_____ Photocopy machine with large print capability
_____ Adjustable lighting with magnification
_____ Other (please specify)

10. *Does staff know how to use all the items checked above?*

11. *Does the library have adapted computer workstations?*

12. *If so, what adaptations do the workstations have? Please check all that you have:*

_____ Wheelchair height table/ carrel
_____ Adjustable height table/ carrel
_____ Screen enlarger device (magnifier)
_____ Text magnification software
_____ Screen reader (voice output software)
_____ Text to speech software (reading software)
_____ Voice recognition system (voice input software)
_____ Thought organization software
_____ Braille printer
_____ Large print printer
_____ Alternate keyboards
_____ Mouse alternatives

_____ Touch screens or overlays
_____ Scanners (OCR)
_____ Switches and switch software
_____ Pointing and typing aids
_____ Other (please specify)

13. *Does staff know how to work all of the checked features?*

14. *Does your library have a webpage? If so, is it accessible? If you are not sure, take the Bobby test at* http://www.cast.org/bobby/

ADDITIONAL QUESTIONS FOR ACADEMIC, SCHOOL, AND SPECIAL LIBRARIES

1. *Do you have reserve collections in alternative formats? Check all that are available.*

     _____ Audio tape
     _____ Computer disk
     _____ Large print
     _____ Braille
     _____ Access to the Perkins School Service
     _____ Other (please specify)

2. *Do you have recommended/ required reading collections in alternative formats? Check all that are available.*

     _____ Audio tape
     _____ Computer disk
     _____ Large print
     _____ Braille
     _____ Access to the Perkins School Service
     _____ Other (please specify)

3. *Is the campus/ school district testing center in your facility? If so, what accommodations are offered for people with disabilities?*

4. *Is there an on campus office that provides services for people with disabilities? If yes, what are the hours of operation?*

5. *Does the campus office for disability services provide any services within the library to library users? If yes, what?*

6. Who provides direct assistance to people with disabilities using the library?
Check all that apply.

     _____ Patron's personal assistant
     _____ Staff from another agency/ department
     _____ Trained volunteers from another agency/ department
     _____ Library staff
     _____ Trained library volunteers

7. What are the hours these assistants are available?

USER and NON-USER SURVEY: PLANNING FOR LIBRARY SERVICES FOR PEOPLE WITH DISABILITIES

Note: This survey is available in alternative formats (braille, audio, and electronic). Please request the version you would like.

1. If you use the library, when did you use it last?

2. In what way(s) does your disability make it difficult to use the library? Check all that apply.

    ____ transportation to library
    ____ parking at library
    ____ physical access to and within building
    ____ hours open
    ____ communication with staff
    ____ attitudes of staff or public
    ____ inability to find or reach library materials
    ____ inability to use library materials
    ____ difficulty using the computers
    ____ other (please specify)

Please continue on the next page.

3. Which library services do you use or would you like to use? Check all that apply.

       ____ information and referral
       ____ check out materials
       ____ read newspapers and magazines
       ____ children's services
       ____ Internet and database searching
       ____ programs and events
       ____ other (please specify)

4. What could the library provide to assist you in using the library's materials and services?

       ____ books by mail
       ____ extended loan periods
       ____ reference services by fax or TTY
       ____ alternative formats of materials (specify)
       ____ different technology (specify)
       ____ help finding books
       ____ other assistance from staff
       ____ other (please specify)

Please continue on the next page.

5. Have you requested these materials/ services in the past? If so, were they provided to you? If not, what reason was given?

___ Yes   ___ No

Reason:

6. Have you ever used a computer or other equipment at the library?

___ Yes   ___ No

7. Did you already know how to use it?

___ Yes   ___ No

8. Were you given instructions or help?

___ Yes   ___ No

9. What could we do to make the computer workstations easier for you to use?

Please continue on the next page.

10. Do you have access to a computer at home or at work?

_____ Yes   _____ No

If so, is it

_____ Macintosh   _____ IBM compatible

11. If you have a computer at home or at work, what adaptive equipment or software do you use?

12. What service agencies besides the library do you use for information and referral?

13. How do you find out about programs and services at the library?

Please continue on the next page.

14. How can the library best communicate with you in the future?

15. What is your disability? (optional)

16. Please mark your age range:

     ____ 6 - 12 years old
     ____ 13- 22
     ____ 23-65
     ____ 66 and older

17. Are you currently in school? If so, at what level?

     ____ Elementary school
     ____ High school
     ____ Community college
     ____ University
     ____ Post graduate

Please continue on the next page.

17. If you have completed your education, please specify the extent of your schooling.

_____ Elementary school
_____ High School
_____ GED
_____ Community college
_____ University
_____ Post graduate degree

18. Are you currently employed?

_____ Yes   _____ No

If yes, _____ Part time   _____ Full time

19. Other comments (please use back of sheet):

Thank you for completing our survey!

PLANNING PROCESS BUDGET WORKSHEET

Category	Number	Unit Cost	Cost
Committee Support			
Photocopies	_____	_____	_____
Braille transcription	_____	_____	_____
Audiorecording	_____	_____	_____
Postage	_____	_____	_____
Other	_____	_____	_____
Meeting Costs			
Room rental	_____	_____	_____
Refreshments	_____	_____	_____
Technology	_____	_____	_____
Interpreter fees	_____	_____	_____
Facilitator fees	_____	_____	_____
Facilitator travel	_____	_____	_____
Other	_____	_____	_____
Staff Costs			
Overtime	_____	_____	_____
Substitutes	_____	_____	_____
Temporaries	_____	_____	_____
Other	_____	_____	_____
Publishing Plan			
Desktop publishing	_____	_____	_____
Graphic artist	_____	_____	_____
Braille transcription	_____	_____	_____
Audio recording	_____	_____	_____
Other	_____	_____	_____
Other	_____	_____	_____
	_____	_____	_____
	_____	_____	_____
	_____	_____	_____
Total			$_____